Occupational Therapy in Oncology and Palliative Care

Occupational Therapy in Oncology and Palliative Care

2nd edition

Edited by
JILL COOPER

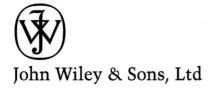

John Wiley & Sons, Ltd

Other Wiley Editorial Offices

John Wiley & Sons Inc., 111 River Street, Hoboken, NJ 07030, USA

Jossey-Bass, 989 Market Street, San Francisco, CA 94103-1741, USA

Wiley-VCH Verlag GmbH, Boschstr. 12, D-69469 Weinheim, Germany

John Wiley & Sons Australia Ltd, 42 McDougall Street, Milton, Queensland 4064, Australia

John Wiley & Sons (Asia) Pte Ltd, 2 Clementi Loop #02-01, Jin Xing Distripark, Singapore 129809

John Wiley & Sons Canada Ltd, 22 Worcester Road, Etobicoke, Ontario, Canada M9W 1L1

Wiley also publishes its books in a variety of electronic formats. Some content that appears in print may not be available in electronic books.

Library of Congress Cataloging-in-Publication Data

Occupational therapy in oncology and palliative care / edited and co-written by Jill Cooper. – 2nd ed.
    p. ; cm.
  Includes bibliographical references and index.
  ISBN-13: 978-0-470-01962-7 (alk. paper)
  ISBN-10: 0-470-01962-X (alk. paper)
  1. Cancer – Palliative treatment. 2. Occupational therapy.
  [DNLM: 1. Neoplasms – therapy. 2. Neoplasms – complications. 3. Occupational Therapy – methods. 4. Palliative Care – methods. QZ 266 O15 2006] I. Cooper, Jill.
  RC271.P33O23 2006
  616.99′406 – dc22

                                            2005030099

A catalogue record for this book is available from the British Library
ISBN-13   978-0-470-01962-7
ISBN-10   0-470-01962-X
Typeset by SNP Best-set Typesetter Ltd., Hong Kong

DEDICATED TO PETER, JOYCE AND STANLEY

Contents

Contributors

Helen Barrett BA (Hons), BSc (Hons), OT
Senior Occupational Therapist, The Royal Marsden NHS Foundation Trust, Downs Road, Sutton, Surrey, UK SM2 5PT

Kathryn Boog BSc (Hons), OT
Senior Occupational Therapist, St Columba's Hospice, Boswall Road, Edinburgh, UK EH5 3RW

Anne Bostock DipCOT, OT
Senior Occupational Therapist, Sue Ryder Care – Leckhampton Court Hospice, Leckhampton Court, Church Road, Leckhampton, Cheltenham, UK GL53 0QJ

Will Chegwidden BSc OT (Hons), OT
Senior Occupational Therapist, The Royal London & St Bartholomew's NHS Trust, London, UK E1

Jill Cooper DipCOT, DMS, OT
Head Occupational Therapist, The Royal Marsden NHS Foundation Trust, Fulham Road, London, UK SW3 6JJ

Derek Doyle MD, OBE
Retired Consultant in Palliative Medicine, Senior Editor of The Oxford Textbook of Palliative Medicine, Vice President and Honorary Vice Chair of the National Council for Palliative Care

Shelley Ellis BSc (Hons), OT
Senior Occupational Therapist, Great Oaks Dean Forest Hospice and community, The Gorse, Coleford, Gloucestershire, UK GL16 8QE

Gail Eva BSc (OT)(Hons), MSc, OT
Team Leader Hospital and Community Palliative Care, Sir Michael Sobell House Hospice, Churchill Hospital, Headington, Oxford, UK OX3 7LJ

Camilla Hawkins DipCOT, LHMC, MScOT, OT
Senior Occupational Therapist, Mildmay Hospital, London, UK E1

Gemma Lindsell BA (Hons), DipCOT, OT
Senior Occupational Therapist, The Royal Marsden NHS Foundation Trust, Fulham Road, London, UK SW3 6JJ

Daniel Lowrie BHSc (OT), OT
Lecturer/practitioner Occupational Therapist, The Royal Marsden NHS Foundation Trust, Fulham Road, London, UK SW3 6JJ

Sara Mathewson BSc(Hons), OT
Senior Occupational Therapist in Palliative Care, Gloucester Royal Hospital NHS Foundation Trust, Great Western Road, Gloucester, UK GL1 3NN

Lilias Methven DipCOT, OT
Senior Occupational Therapist, Gloucester Royal Hospital NHS Foundation Trust, Great Western Road, Gloucester, UK GL1 3NN

Claire Tester DipCOT, PGDip, OT
Senior Occupational Therapist, Rachel House Children's Hospice, Avenue Road, Kinross, UK KY13 8FX

Julie Watterson BSc (Hons), OT
Senior Occupational Therapist, Prospect Hospice, Moormead Road, Wroughton, Swindon, Wilts, UK SN4 9BY

Foreword

The death of Dame Cicely Saunders (in July 2005), the charismatic visionary behind the Hospice Movement, brought home to many of us both the importance of what she advocated and the remarkable, worldwide acceptance of the principles of palliative care. From modest beginnings in 1967 there are now, in 2005, more than 8000 palliative care services worldwide, more than 20 academic professorial chairs, countless undergraduate and postgraduate qualifications available, and more than 300 multiprofessional research projects on the go at any one time. In the United Kingdom alone there are 217 in-patient palliative care units, 356 community palliative care services, 258 day care units and 83 hospital palliative care teams.

At the heart of each one, whatever the type of service, are the patients and their loved ones. Each hopes for cure or if cure is unrealistic, for a life worth living, a life that they and they alone can say has 'quality'. It may not be a long life, any more than it might resemble their life before their illness but, for them, it is a life worth living – a life with as little dependency on others as possible, a life without suffering, a life with smiles and happy times shared with family and friends preferably in their own homes.

Palliative care provision has burgeoned, as we have seen, but it has changed in other ways since the first edition of this book. No longer is it primarily concerned with oncology patients. Today hospital palliative care teams can expect to be invited to see patients with advanced cardiac, respiratory, neurological and even infectious conditions. No longer will most be in the far advanced stages of illness. Some may still be under their care a year or more later, still spending much of their time at home.

Oncology has changed, almost as dramatically as has palliative care. With earlier referrals, more sophisticated investigations and new drugs many malignancies can be controlled for years – not cured but controlled sufficiently for patients and carers to have every reason to talk about quality rather than quantity of life. No longer is there a false dichotomy between oncology care and palliative care as was once the case. Oncology teams now offer good palliative care and see that as part and parcel of their work. The two disciplines for whom this book is written now recognize that neither can work in isolation, that they share aims and many skills, and that they can and must work together respecting the training, the skills and the contributions of the other.

The society in which we live and work is also changing, perhaps quicker and more radically than many of us would wish. No matter how much people say that when the time comes they would like to die at home, studies are showing that this is seldom achieved. No matter how much family doctors and community nurses would like to care for the terminally ill at home, this is becoming ever more difficult because of their workload, inadequate resources, and unsatisfactory out-of-hours cover. Cover of the chronically ill and aged is suffering. Resources for care, whatever the condition, are being directed more towards cure than long term or palliative care. 'Hard' research attracts more funding than 'soft' research into such things as feelings, spiritual needs, needs of relatives, stress of the carers and quality of life. Some would go so far as to say that since the first edition of this book we have moved back to being more interested in the pathology than in the person with that pathology, vehemently as most would deny that.

What cannot be denied is that occupational therapy has grown as a discipline and grown in importance and is certain to continue on that road. It is not an optional extra in today's care team, whether in hospital or community. Today, the occupational therapist is an indispensable, integral member of each team but the value of her/his contribution will largely rest on the adequacy of her training, her well-informed understanding of the work and contributions of other disciplines, and sensitivity to the nature of changes in our society. The challenges of this work are truly enormous but so too are the rewards.

I commend this new edition as a major contribution to better care for people at one of the most frightening times of life. No greater challenge and no greater rewards can any of us ever have than caring for those on their final, often very long and lonely, road of life.

Dr Derek Doyle
Hon. Vice Chairman National Council for Palliative Care
July 2005

Preface

The second edition of this book aims to explore further occupational therapy for persons with life-threatening and life-limiting illnesses. The most common diseases that most occupational therapists will encounter are cancer and heart disease, as well as other conditions, which are classified under the umbrella term of palliative care, such as HIV/AIDS, neurological and congenital illnesses. The fundamental principles of occupational therapy in oncology and palliative care still apply and this edition will discuss and examine treatment programmes and approaches that have been developed with evidence-based practice.

Specific solutions may still not exist for all specific problems. Individual coping mechanisms are required for people whether they have physical, psychological or psychosocial difficulties so the occupational therapist needs to refine their core and problem-solving skills and analyse each case as it arises.

Working with individuals who have cancer or are at the palliative stages of a disease involves considering their ability to survive and, if the illness is terminal, assessing how to facilitate them and their carers in achieving optimum quality of life in their remaining time. This second edition focuses on suggested occupational therapy interventions that can be adapted to suit different work settings and environments.

The first chapter revisits the basic terminology for cancer and palliative care interventions, treatments, side effects and related issues. This is followed by a discussion of the principles of occupational therapy in this clinical area, first in general terms and then with specific reference to more complex issues. Subsequent chapters discuss more specific symptoms and approaches as well as exploring the use of creativity as a psychodynamic activity and examining palliative care far more broadly, particularly in paediatrics. The examples of treatment programmes are a consensus of expert practitioners throughout the UK and are designed to be used and adapted to suit individual requirements, work settings and requirements.

This second edition aims to underpin clinical practice with evidence-based information wherever possible and should be used to support practice development and used as a workbook format. In some scenarios, the individuals receiving treatment are referred to as clients; at other times, they are referred to as patients. This depends on the health care setting.

Various political influences, particularly in the United Kingdom, have occurred since the publication of the first edition in 1997 including the NHS

Cancer Plan (DoH, 2000) and NICE Guidelines for Supportive and Palliative Care (NICE, 2004) and these continue to recognize the value of occupational therapy in this clinical area.

Jill Cooper
Royal Marsden NHS Foundation Trust

REFERENCES

DoH (2000) *The NHS Cancer Plan: A plan for investment, a plan for reform*, Department of Health, London.
NICE (2004) *Improving Supportive and Palliative Care for Adults with Cancer: The Manual*, National Institute for Clinical Excellence, London.

ACKNOWLEDGEMENTS

I wish to thank the following for permission to use copyright material:

- Bloomsbury Publishing plc for Figure 1.1: 'Common symptoms and signs of cancer' reproduced here in Chapter 1. Tobias, J. and Eaton, K. (2001) *Living with Cancer*, Bloomsbury, London.
- M.A. Healthcare Ltd for Figure 2.1: 'Breakdown of all occupational therapy activity' reproduced here in Chapter 2. Cooper, J. and Littlechild, B. (2004) *International Journal of Therapy and Rehabilitation*, **11**(7).
- College of Occupational Therapists for extract from HOPE (2004) *Occupational Therapy Intervention in Cancer*, College of Occupational Therapists, London, reproduced here in Chapter 3.
- Elsevier Limited for extract from Oliver, K. and Sewell, L. (2002) in *Occupational Therapy and Physical Dysfunction*, 5th edn (eds. A. Turner, M. Foster and S.E. Johnson), Churchill Livingstone, Edinburgh, reproduced here in Chapter 5.
- Oxford University Press for Figure 8.1: 'Model of curative and palliative care relationships' reproduced here in Chapter 8. Goldman, A. and Schuller, I. (2001) *Palliative Care for Non-cancer Patients* (eds J. Addington-Hall and J. Higginson), Oxford University Press, Oxford.

I would also like to thank:

- the staff and patients of The Royal Marsden NHS Foundation Trust, with whom it is always a pleasure and honour to work;
- my fellow occupational therapists in HOPE (Occupational Therapy Specialist Section in HIV/AIDS, Oncology, Palliative Care and Education) with whom I am very proud to have worked on various projects.

I wish to thank specifically:

- Helen Barrett, Phil Canning, Charlie Ewer-Smith, Chervonne Hopkinson, Gemma Lindsell, Daniel Lowrie, Andrea Mitchell, Sarah Patterson, Astrid van Dijken, Jo Bray and Barbara Littlechild, all of whom have contributed so much to various subjects covered in this book.

In addition, I wish to thank:

- Kathy Thompson, Nicki Thompson, Diane Strange, Paul Armitage, Gill Skilton and Douglas Guerrero for their kind support and help in specific areas. Also Steve Park, Assistant Professor of Occupational Therapy at Pacific University, Oregon, for the information drawn from his lectures 1998–1999 used in Chapter 13.

Introduction

This edition refers to occupational therapy in the treatment of conditions such as cancer and others requiring palliative care and also aims to encompass other illnesses than cancer that result in a chronic debilitating condition or non-curable disease and which might be life-threatening. The occupational therapist assesses and analyses functional problems in any illness irrespective of the origin of the disease, but it is the diagnosis and prognosis that affects the intervention and urgency with which the occupational therapy service is needed. Occupational therapists aim to maintain the people whom they are treating at their optimum independence and quality of life. This is carried out preferably in their own homes by controlling symptoms and providing home-care support together with training for the carers. Intervention occurs from the early stages of health promotion to the more advanced stages when disability and illness have become more severe and chronic. A holistic, client-centred approach is needed, which is constantly reassessed according to the needs of the individuals and their carers. The fundamental areas in which occupational therapy contributes include:

- assisting clients with activities for the treatment of physical dysfunction;
- retraining clients in personal and domestic activities that are necessary for daily living;
- assessing seating needs and prescribing wheelchairs and pressure relieving cushions;
- retraining clients in order to help them with cognitive and perceptual dysfunction;
- splinting to prevent deformities and control pain;
- making home assessments;
- referring to and liaising with social services for ongoing home assessment and provision of equipment;
- helping with lifestyle management including investigating hobbies and leisure pursuits;
- providing advice on and education about relaxation techniques;
- aiding breathlessness management;
- aiding management of fatigue and energy conservation;

- providing support and education for carers;
- assisting with psychological adjustment and goal-setting related to loss of function.

In order to establish rapport and introduce the occupational therapy service to clients, the occupational therapist can make them aware of the services that are available, even if those services are not required immediately. If clients know what is available and where to obtain it they can make use of appropriate services at a later date as and when necessary. This avoids needless struggle and avoids the occupational therapy intervention occurring at a time of crisis, when it could be called upon earlier, thus preventing the crisis from happening.

As the assessment of each client covers many aspects of life it is necessary for an occupational therapist to establish a good rapport with the individual. Even the simplest of interactions can raise numerous issues. It may be that all the occupational therapist does is provide a padded bathboard to help an individual wash comfortably. The ramifications of this include:

- giving clients the choice of when to bathe rather than them having to wait for a carer;
- reducing anxiety;
- promoting self-esteem;
- maintaining dignity
- enabling privacy
- avoiding being dependent on others;
- providing safety.

The range of services available to individuals with cancer, or any life-threatening illness, continues to change dramatically and there is now firm emphasis on multiprofessional teamwork rather than on medical and nursing staff alone. Occupational therapy is one part of the service provided by the multiprofessional team and it relies on early referral, ongoing communication and liaison and support for all its members if it is to work efficiently and effectively. In particular, the entire team needs to be aware of the changing needs of the individual as the disease progresses.

The multiprofessional team in oncology and palliative care is likely to comprise:

Occupational therapist	Nursing staff
Physiotherapist	Dietitian
Speech and language therapist	Pastoral care
Community liaison	Surgical appliance officer
Home-care nurse	Art therapist
Social worker	Medical staff
Psychological medicine	

The National Council for Hospice and Specialist Palliative Care Services (2000) states that: 'effective rehabilitation is achieved through the work of a well-integrated team of professionals from different disciplines.' Team members must develop an understanding of each other's roles within the team. There will inevitably be some overlap and blurring of roles if team members are working closely together, and if members are sensitive to patients' needs to deal with key individuals. The most important members of the team are the patients, their family and carers.

Occupational therapists find that defining their own role clearly helps them cope with working with the acutely or terminally ill. It should, however, be borne in mind that while clear role identification enables health care workers to achieve their goals, this should not prevent people from working together where boundaries overlap and complement each other.

Providers of oncological and palliative care are increasingly employing occupational therapy services as there is greater emphasis on supporting individuals in their own homes. Occupational therapists have taken the initiative to develop networking and communication within the profession by establishing the Specialist Section of HOPE (Occupational therapists working in HIV/AIDS, Oncology and Palliative Care Education). This, together with growing numbers of palliative care modules in postgraduate education, indicates a rising need for occupational therapists and the expansion of education in these areas.

REFERENCE

National Council for Hospice and Specialist Palliative Care Services (2000) *Fulfilling Lives. Rehabilitation in Palliative Care*, Land and Unwin Ltd, Northamptonshire.

1 What is Cancer?

JILL COOPER

Cancer is a general term applied to tumours or growths. The terms oncology, anaplasia, neoplasms may all be used as an alternative to the word cancer. Body cells normally regenerate and die continually so the number of cells remains constant. Cancer is the disordered and uncontrolled growth of cells within a specific organ or tissue type. If left untreated, they grow steadily resulting in a mass, tumour or growth. The tumour may be benign or malignant. Benign tumours grow slowly and do not recur after excision. They can still be life-threatening if untreated as they can affect vital organs. They are usually curable if they are treated early.

The human body is made up of 10 trillion cells (Knight, 2004), and there are over 100 different types of cells. 25 million cells are replaced every second in adult life. All cells replicate themselves, usually 50–60 times before cell death. Malignant cells grow in an irregular pattern (Gabriel, 2004, p. 4). The smallest detectable tumour is approximately 1 cm in diameter and already contains 1 billion cells. Normal cells know when to grow, to specialize (differentiate), to die (apoptosis), to release certain products or proteins needed by other cells to grow and how to build complex tissue structures.

Cancer is not a single disease but a complex sequence of events (Haylock, 1998). Cancers not only develop at a single site, but also result from malignant change within a single clone, or cluster, of cells. This then multiplies and acquires different changes that give it a survival chance over its neighbours. Cancer cells develop when they have defects in regulation that govern normal cell proliferation and homeostasis, i.e. they lose the ability to die and continue to multiply.

Tobias and Eaton (2001) describe how several steps are required before a normal cell becomes a malignant one. Cell growth and division is profoundly influenced by the presence of critical genes. Oncogenes drive the cell towards malignancy and suppressor genes mutate and result in a loss of normal regulatory or restraining function.

Woodhouse *et al.* (1997) describe the process by which cancer cells spread or metastasize:

Occupational Therapy in Oncology and Palliative Care. Edited by J. Cooper
© 2006 John Wiley & Sons Ltd

- angiogenesis: the generation of blood vessels around the primary tumour that increases the chances for tumour cells to reach the blood stream and colonize in secondary sites;
- attachment or adhesion: tumour cells need to attach themselves to other cells and/or cell matrix proteins;
- invasion: tumour cells move across the normal barriers imposed by the extracellular matrix;
- tumour cell proliferation: new colony of tumour cells is stimulated to grow at a secondary site.

Malignant tumours, therefore, infiltrate and destroy the normal tissues surrounding them and spread to other sites either by blood or the lymphatic system. These are then called metastases or secondaries.

Although terminal and palliative care are phrases often used interchangeably, terminal actually refers to individuals who are actively dying so likely to be in the last few days of life. A diagnosis of cancer does not necessarily mean that the disease will become terminal and the phrase terminal illness can refer equally well to the end stages of neurological, viral or respiratory illness.

Palliation refers to the alleviation of symptoms rather than the attempt to cure disease and it is associated with the advanced stages of all diseases including cancer and HIV/AIDS. The World Health Organization (WHO) (1990) defines palliative care as 'the active total care of patients and their families by a multiprofessional team when the patient's disease is no longer responsive to curative treatment.' In occupational therapy there is not a finite point between acute and palliative care. The focus may change from one to the other as the client progresses or deteriorates. Symptoms are approached in a similar manner and treatment depends on the client's functional status. Dysfunction may be the result of the tumour and/or side-effects of medical intervention such as chemotherapy, radiotherapy or surgery.

CLASSIFICATION OF TUMOURS

Tumours are classified according to histogenesis – the tissues and cells where they originate. Cancers are often described in terms of degrees of differentiation. The tumour's degree of differentiation is the extent to which it resembles the normal tissue from which it is derived. If it closely resembles the normal tissue it is well differentiated, otherwise it is poorly differentiated. When tumour cells lose all similarity to the corresponding normal tissue, they are referred to as undifferentiated or anaplastic. Tumours of the muscle and connective tumours are classified as in Table 1.1.

Table 1.1 Nomenclature of connective tissue and muscle tumours

Tissue of origin	Benign tumours	Malignant tumours
Fibrous tissue	Fibroma	Fibrosarcoma
Adipose (fatty) tissue	Lipoma	Liposarcoma
Bone	Osteoma	Osteosarcoma
Cartilage	Chondroma	Chondrosarcoma
Connective tissue near joints	Benign synovioma	Synovial sarcoma
Blood vessel endothelium	Haemangioma	Haemangiosarcoma
Lymph vessel endothelium	Lymphangioma	Lymphangiosarcoma
Smooth muscle	Leiomyoma	Leiomyosarcoma
Striated muscle	Rhabdomyoma	Rhabdomyosarcoma

(From Gowing and Fisher (1989) cited in Cooper (1997))

INCIDENCE

The incidence of cancer is increasing possibly due to lifestyle and the increasing age of the population (Gabriel, 2004, p. 11). There are 1:250 men and 1:300 women diagnosed as suffering from cancer every year (Souhami and Tobias, 2003). As the elderly population grows and as more people with cancer live longer due to better treatment, there are increasing numbers of people with residual dysfunction and disabilities who require occupational therapy. Although the treatment and management of the primary tumour have obviously been the main focus of medical input, metastatic spread is still the main cause of death (Woodhouse *et al.*, 1997). This spread often develops before diagnosis and treatment have begun, so prognosis is not altered by treatment of the primary cancer.

The highest recorded incidences of cancers in females in England in 2002 are breast, lung and colorectal cancers. Those in males are prostate, lung and colorectal cancers (Office for National Statistics, 2005). Early intervention with cancer treatment invariably has a better chance of survival.

AETIOLOGICAL FACTORS

In many types of cancer there is still no clear evidence of what triggers the initial malignant change. Some factors are known: they are listed in Table 1.2.

Diet is emerging as an increasingly important risk factor for lower bowel cancers.

Table 1.2 Aetiology of cancer

Ionizing radiation	
Atomic bomb and nuclear accidents	Acute leukaemia and breast cancer
X-rays	Acute leukaemia, squamous cell skin carcinoma
Ultraviolet irradiation	Basal cell carcinoma, squamous cell skin carcinomas, melanoma
Background irradiation	Acute leukaemia
Inhaled or ingested carcinogens	
Atmospheric pollution with polycytic hydrocarbons	Lung cancer
Cigarette smoking	Lung cancer, laryngeal cancer, bladder cancer
Asbestos	Mesothelioma, bronchial carcinoma, lung cancer
Arsenic	Lung cancer, skin cancer
Aluminium	Bladder cancer
Aromatic amines	Bladder cancer
Benzene	Erythroleukaemia
Polyvinyl chloride	Angiosarcoma of the liver

(From Cooper 1997)

SYMPTOMS

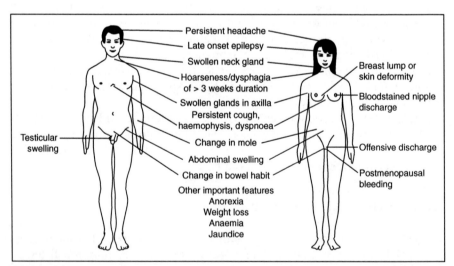

(From Tobias and Eaton 2001. Reproduced by kind permission of Bloomsbury Publishing plc)

Figure 1.1 Common symptoms and signs of cancer

INVESTIGATIONS

SCREENING

Breast and cervical cancer screening is well established; breast cancer screening is only certain for females aged over 50 years. Cervical screening programmes are offered as often as resources allow. Trials have failed to show efficacy for lung cancer screening, and testicular cancer has such a good cure rate that screening could only enhance prognosis.

STAGING

Staging identifies the stage that the disease has reached and is one way of establishing the factors that are likely to influence prognosis in any individual. The TNM system evaluates the tumour by size, lymph node spread and presence of distance metastases:

T – tumour size, site and depth of the primary tumour's invasion depending on the type of tumour, evaluated on a scale ranging from T1–T5;

N – lymph node spread, evaluated on a scale ranging from N1–N5;

M – the presence of distance metastases, evaluated on a scale ranging from M1–M5;

e.g. T3, N1, M0 laryngeal cancer implies a primary tumour sufficiently locally advanced to have affixed the vocal cord and early lymph node invasion causing a palpable swelling in the neck but no evidence of metastatic spread.

OTHER INVESTIGATIONS

The individual undergoes many of the following investigations in order for diagnosis and treatment procedures to be established:

- x-ray
- blood counts
- enzymes
- ultrasound
- computed tomography (CT) scan
- positron emission tomography (PET) scan
- magnetic resonance imaging (MRI) scan
- isotope scanning
- surgery.

TREATMENTS/INTERVENTIONS

SURGERY

Cancer surgery is classified as:

- diagnostic and staging – biopsy taken. Primarily curative, where local control of cancer is essential as the primary site either causes or contributes substantially towards death;
- adjuvant – used alongside chemotherapy and/or radiotherapy;
- prophylactic – laser surgery to remove premalignant cells and preventing further tumour growth;
- reconstructive – to rebuild areas removed by other surgery;
- palliative – used in symptom control if a tumour compresses other areas or a nerve block is required for pain control;
- emergency – to remove a life-threatening obstruction;
- surgery for metastases;
- surgery for vascular access – insertion of Hickman line (central intravenous line) in the superior vena cava or right atrium through which chemotherapy can be given. Also insertion of feeding gastrostomy;
- laser surgery.

RADIOTHERAPY

Radiotherapy is the use of ionizing radiation to destroy cancer cells. The aim is to destroy or inactivate cancer cells while preserving the integrity of normal tissues within the treatment field. It is often able to control the tumour with minimal physiological disturbance. There are different types of radiotherapy, and these should be matched to the individual's diagnosis and needs. The factors taken into account when planning radiotherapy include the type and stage of tumour, localization of tumour and adjacent normal structures.

Detailed planning is needed and this may include the preparation of an individually moulded cast. The individual wears this during radiotherapy and it positions him or her correctly. The exact positioning and dosage of radiotherapy is calculated. Radiographers position the individual on the couch, using marks made on the skin in indelible ink, and the radiation beam is switched on. Radiographers or radiotherapists observe the individual via a window or closed-circuit TV in the treatment area, using an intercom for communication.

Radiotherapy is used alone or adjuvant to surgery and/or chemotherapy. In addition to treating localized tumours it is often used as a palliative treatment to relieve pain or bleeding, or to suppress bone metastases which are developing into pathological fractures. Side-effects may include:

- fatigue and malaise, sometimes caused by bone marrow depression;
- anorexia, nausea and vomiting;

- alopecia;
- inflammation around the site being treated, causing internal side-effects such as mucositis, oesophagitis, laryngitis, diarrhoea, cystitis;
- anxiety and altered body image.

CHEMOTHERAPY

Chemotherapy is the use of cytotoxic (cell poisoning) drugs to kill cancer cells. The drugs enter the bloodstream and destroy cancer cells by interfering with the cells' ability to grow and divide. Although normal cells can be damaged, most healthy tissue grows back again.

Chemotherapy can be used in the following ways:

- neo-adjuvant – given prior to surgery to shrink the tumour with the aim of making surgery easier as there is less tumour and increased likelihood of cure;
- adjuvant – in combination with radiotherapy or surgery to eliminate micrometastases and increase the likelihood of cure in some cancers;
- primary or curative – given on its own or in combination with other modalities with the aim of eradicating all tumour cells;
- palliative – aims to improve quality of life though not necessarily increase life expectancy.

Methods of administration:

- oral
- intravenous/intra-arterial
- intramuscular/subcutaneous
- intracavity
- intrathecal
- intralesion
- topical.

Most cytotoxic drugs are toxic to bone marrow so lower the blood cell count. Blood tests are carried out regularly to ensure the individual is strong enough to cope. When very high dose chemotherapy is given, bone marrow is taken from the client before treatment and returned later so the marrow is not affected by the drug.

Short-term side-effects may include:

- hair loss
- nausea and vomiting
- constipation or diarrhoea
- stomatitis, cystitis
- pain at tumour site or jaw

- fatigue, flu-like symptoms.

Long-term side-effects may include

- bone marrow suppression
- alopecia, skin reactions, nail ridging
- fatigue
- sexual function – infertility, loss of libido
- neurological problems – neuropathy, hearing loss
- organ damage – liver, cardiac, renal, lung.

HORMONE THERAPY

Hormone therapy is less widely used than chemotherapy and often seen as the gentler alternative. Its indications are limited as only a small minority of tumours are hormone sensitive. Breast and prostate cancers, for example, are responsive. It has fewer side-effects than chemotherapy and is more durable.

BONE MARROW TRANSPLANTATION (BMT)

Bone marrow transplantation aims to eradicate deficient or malignant bone marrow. Originally used for treatment of leukaemia, it is now more widely used to increase dose intensity with an acceptable margin of safety.

Allogenic transplantation – the donor and the recipient are matched, often from a sibling. The individual undergoes very intensive chemotherapy to ablate bone marrow and the transplant repopulates the recipient's marrow.

Autologous transplantation – the individual's own marrow is removed, and replaced after high-dose chemotherapy.

Blood stem cell transplantation – the individual's bone marrow is stimulated by low-dose chemotherapy to liberate early marrow precursor cells into the circulating blood. The marrow is collected, concentrated and used as support for high-dose chemotherapy. Much higher doses of chemotherapy can be given safely.

BMT is used to treat:

- Acute myeloid leukaemia (AML)
- Acute lymphoblastic leukaemia (ALL)
- Chronic myeloid leukaemia (CML)
- Neuroblastoma
- In severe immune deficiency states, thalassaemia major and sickle cell anaemia.

Individuals treated with BMT become extremely tired and weak and may undergo a period of isolation while the body is immunosuppressed.

ACTION POINTS

1. Using websites and the literature available, collate a profile of common cancers including the aetiology, incidence and prevalence, treatments, symptoms and side-effects. Consider the functional difficulties that the sufferers might have.
2. Choose a specific diagnosis with a given individual, decide on age, marital status, etc., and explore the primary investigations through to the potential long-term issues and what impact these would have on an individual's independence.
3. Compare the occupational therapy input with individuals undergoing acute care with that of individuals who are nearing the end of treatment.

REFERENCES

Cooper, J. (1997) *Occupational Therapy in Oncology and Palliative Care*, Whurr, London.

Gabriel, J. (2004) *The Biology of Cancer*, Whurr, London.

Gowing, N. and Fisher, C. (1989) The general pathology of tumours, in *Oncology for Nurses and Health Care Professionals* (ed. R. Tiffany), Harper & Row, Beaconsfield.

Haylock, P. J. (1998) Cancer metastasis: An update, *Seminars in Oncology Nursing*, **14**(3), 172–7.

Knight, L. A. (2004) The cell, in *The Biology of Cancer* (ed. J. Gabriel), Whurr, London.

Office for National Statistics (2005) Cancer. *National Statistics Online*: www.statistics.gov.uk accessed July 2005.

Souhami, R. and Tobias, J. (2003) *Cancer and its Management*, 4th edn, Blackwell Science, Oxford.

Tobias, J. and Eaton, K. (2001) *Living with Cancer*, Bloomsbury, London.

Woodhouse, E. C., Chuaqui, R. F. and Liotta, L. A. (1997) General mechanisms of metastasis, *Cancer* **80**(8 Suppl), 1529–37.

World Health Organization (1990) World Health Organization Definition of Palliative Care: www.who.int/hiv/topics/palliative/PalliativeCare/en accessed July 2005.

RECOMMENDED READING

Armstrong, L. (2001) *It's Not About the Bike: My journey back to life*, Yellow Jersey Press, London.

Diamond, J. (1998) *'C' Because Cowards Get Cancer Too*, Vermillion, London.

Gabriel, J. (2004) *The Biology of Cancer*, Whurr, London.

King, R. (2000) *Cancer Biology*, Prentice Hall, London.

Souhami, R. and Tobias, J. (2003) *Cancer and its Management*, 4th edn, Blackwell Science, Oxford.

Tobias, J. and Eaton, K. (2001) *Living with Cancer*, Bloomsbury, London.
WHO (1990) World Health Organization Definition of Palliative Care.

www.who.int/hiv/topics/palliative/PalliativeCare/en
www.doh.gov.uk/cancer
www.cancerresearchuk.org
www.statistics.gov.uk

2 Challenges Faced by Occupational Therapists in Oncology and Palliative Care

JILL COOPER

Occupational therapists working with people who are terminally ill potentially face a contradiction between the principles and assumptions of rehabilitation-oriented practice and the needs and experiences of clients who are dying (Bye, 1998). It is this contradiction which may confuse the concept of rehabilitation within this clinical field.

Watterson *et al.* (2004) reported on the increasing emphasis on the importance of rehabilitation for individuals with cancer regardless of their prognosis. For rehabilitation to be meaningful and holistic and for optimal outcomes to occur, it is essential for occupational therapists to be client-led in their approach (Law *et al.*, 1995). This in itself is not a dilemma for occupational therapists because they use this approach in all areas of practice, but clients with terminal illness may initially present occupational therapists with no tangible improvements in functional ability, possibly leading to therapists losing self-confidence in their skills (Bennett, 1991). Occupational therapists need to have insight into their own needs. Appendix 1 explores how to deal with working with people who are potentially dying, more specifically the bereavement caused (Gordon, personal communication, 1995). Appendix 2 looks at factors influencing whether or not staff cope when working in potentially stressful situations (Faulkner and Maguire, 1994).

EXPLORING SELF-MOTIVATION

Occupational therapists should ask themselves why they choose to work with people with a potentially life-threatening illness (Cooper, 1997).

- Is it to fulfil a personal need?
- Is it because I want to be adored by my clients and others?
- What do I put in and what do I get out?

Occupational Therapy in Oncology and Palliative Care. Edited by J. Cooper
© 2006 John Wiley & Sons Ltd

- Which areas do I find most stressful to me personally?
- How do I deal with these?

Potential areas of stress and burnout may include:

- focusing on the person with cancer;
- communication;
- breaking bad news;
- time management, including supervision and notewriting;
- conflict;
- loss;
- grief;
- cultural issues;
- spirituality.

FOCUSING CARE ON THE PERSON WITH CANCER

Various definitions exist regarding patient or client-centred care, with little consensus regarding its exact meaning (Mead and Bower, 2000). It is generally accepted that client-centred care involves the occupational therapist actively listening, encouraging the person with cancer to express wishes and goals, and showing empathy to hear and understand the patient's expectations of the service and points of view. Overall it involves working together with that person regarding the management of occupational therapy.

COMMUNICATION

Poor communication can cause enormous damage to the trust between the person receiving the service and health care professionals. Communication extends beyond verbal and non-verbal communication; the Royal Society of Medicine (2000) reported that the most common complaints made by people with cancer were about poor communication and inadequate information. Its report advised that health professionals needed to know how best to elicit patients' needs and readiness for information as well as their desire for involvement in decision-making. This is not just for medical staff but for all those responsible for care-giving, particularly when occupational therapists claim that their intervention is client-led and client-centred. The report stated that 'patients cannot express informed preference about their care, choose to be involved in decision-making, or indeed choose not to participate, unless they are given sufficient and appropriate information' (Royal Society of Medicine, 2000).

Coulter *et al.* (1999) described how information is required for different purposes such as understanding the presenting symptoms and/or disease, learning about available services, and participating in decisions about treatment options. Information can be provided in various ways. Individuals cannot express informed preferences about their care, or choose to be involved (or not) in shared decision-making unless they are given sufficient and appropriate information. Smith (2000) found that persons with cancer reported a lack of information although theoretically a great deal should have been available.

It is vital that written advice is given to back up verbal discussions as individuals and their carers can only retain a small amount of information at such stressful times. Occupational therapists can produce simple information packages and aides-mémoires for individuals who use the service regarding all aspects of intervention.

Both *The NHS Cancer Plan* (Department of Health, 2000) and the *Cancer Information Strategy* (NHS Executive, 2000) discuss communication and the provision of good quality materials. The Royal Society of Medicine (2000) concluded that health professionals were also likely to need training and support if the patients' information needs were to be met. Key issues included placing a higher priority on patient information, understanding the patients' needs and preferences, and helping the patients to access and understand relevant and appropriate information.

Communication aims to reduce uncertainty, encourage good working relationships and give the client and carers a positive direction in which to move (Cooper, 1997). Non-verbal communication is also essential when working with people who have cancer or who are receiving palliative care. This includes facial expression, eye contact, posture, body language, pitch, pace of voice and touch. Above all, it means giving that person the time to listen, hear their story and acknowledge that you have heard what they are saying.

Communication with other health professionals is essential to ensure seamless service and continuity of care. The person with a life-limiting illness does not have the time or energy to become involved in professional boundary problems. These issues need to be addressed, communicated with the team and resolved if an effective team is to provide the appropriate and effective service.

Occupational therapists also have to challenge themselves about how they communicate:

- Do we hide behind jargon or physically sit behind a desk or table when talking to them?
- Do we stand over the patient rather than sitting and making eye contact at their level while talking to them?
- Do we focus on our agendas to make the job easier for us rather than really look at what they want?

Handouts to accompany treatment sessions can be useful but only if they are explained, appropriate and there is a clear contact name and number for the service. The individuals and their carers can become overwhelmed with too many leaflets, booklets, catalogues and pieces of paper. Occupational therapists should have a range of easy-to-read handouts for their service. They may range from those that explain the safe and appropriate use of equipment, which should accompany equipment when it is provided, to small booklets that cover safe use and manoeuvring of wheelchairs, for example. Other topics from energy conservation to joint protection are widely available in occupational therapy departments. Handouts regarding any intervention should be provided only to complement a treatment session. It is vital that they are not just handed out instead of an assessment and without the professional support as there must be an occupational therapist available to answer the questions that will arise from this information.

It is relatively rare for a patient to completely deny illness, though this could be the individual's coping mechanism. Appendix 3 recommends strategies for communication in interviews (Brewin, 1991).

BREAKING BAD NEWS

Communication skills are paramount in handling bad news. Although the occupational therapist is unlikely to be giving the actual diagnosis of disease or illness, bad news may have to be given regarding future rehabilitation potential, or whether or not a service or item of equipment is available.

The patient should always have hope for a positive future, but the occupational therapist must still deal with information honestly and constructively. Empathy is entirely appropriate and breaking down information may help in giving it. If the occupational therapist is discussing future possibilities with a person with a deteriorating condition, it is acceptable to say 'I wish I had better news but I am afraid. . . .' and discuss the options that are available. Even though patients may not want to accept any of the available options, this is their choice and, if the occupational therapist does not have anything else to suggest, then this needs to be confirmed as honestly and gently as possible.

The opportunity should always be given to talk and think about the situation and how the individual feels, and the occupational therapist should acknowledge these feelings. Patients need individual intervention and are likely to need to be addressed uniquely. However, the occupational therapist can build on their communication skills from experience with other patients.

In the event of families and carers wanting health professionals to collude in keeping information from the actual individual with cancer or other disease, Kaye (1994) advises that health professionals ask each of the persons involved what their understanding of the illness or disease is, and try to address their misconceptions, fears and worries. Glass and Cluxton (2004) state that health-care professionals have an ethical obligation to tell patients and families the truth about their illness, prognosis and available treatment options, including hospice care. Failure to provide truthful information impedes patients and families from making treatment and/or end-of-life choices that are consistent with their wishes. Fear of taking away a patient's hope is a common reason why healthcare professionals may not tell patients the truth about their prognosis. However, this reason is based on misconceptions about hope.

Acknowledging how people feel about receiving bad news gives them the opportunity to reflect on their feelings. Although this can be uncomfortable and very time consuming, this investment in time will help in resolving the difficulties and prevent further difficulties in the future.

TIME MANAGEMENT

Good time management is as essential in coping strategies as any other aspect of the occupational therapy skill base. Cooper and Littlechild (2004) described the range of interventions carried out by a group of occupational therapists working in oncology and palliative care. This study was in a specific geographical area over a specific length of time and was broken down into non-patient as well as patient-related activities (Figure 2.1).

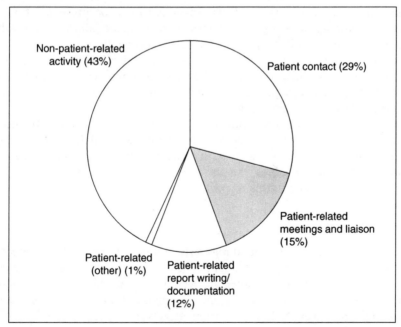

(From Cooper and Littlechild, 2004. Reproduced by kind permission of M.A. Healthcare Ltd.)

Figure 2.1 Breakdown of all occupational therapy activity

The occupational therapist needs to organize the available working hours realistically, to vary the type and amount of client contact, to make a clear distinction between work and personal life and to look after his or her own health and leisure needs (Gamage *et al.*, 1976). No healthcare professional can take on an infinite amount of work. Section 3.2.5 of the College of Occupational Therapists' *Code of Ethics and Professional Conduct* (2005) states that, 'If occupational therapists feel unable to reach the minimum standards determined in 3.2.4, the appropriate manager shall be notified in writing with a copy to the client and referrer, if applicable.'

SUPERVISION

There are various models of supervision used by healthcare professionals and clinical supervision varies amongst occupational therapists. If direct supervision is not available for staff who are lone workers within a palliative care setting, the occupational therapist is obliged to seek a mentor or supervisor from other colleagues.

Team members may choose to present case studies and use peer-group feedback for support and reflection. Occupational therapists who are not being directly supervised should try to talk through problems with trust, confidentiality and objectivity. These sessions should be protected time in which no interruptions, e.g. telephones or bleeps, are allowed and value should be placed on adhering to the supervision time.

Debriefing sessions can be very supportive as they allow the occupational therapist the opportunity to reflect on how circumstances were handled. They also allow those giving support or feedback to discuss alternative options and to consider how the occupational therapist feels.

Exposure to loss and bereavement needs to be acknowledged by the occupational therapist in order for them to deal with its cumulative effects. Individuals cope with loss, and react to it, in different ways. It does not necessarily demand additional resources, but the supervisor needs to be aware of, and sensitive to, staff needs in this respect.

NOTE WRITING

Patient notes must be maintained regularly. It is easy to neglect this aspect of work when one has a busy caseload, but it is essential to incorporate time into treatment sessions to ensure notes are written up and this must be adhered to strictly. The College of Occupational Therapists' *Code of Ethics and Professional Conduct* (2005) legal requirements governing occupational therapy records and documentation state that:

3.3.1 Every client shall have a clearly recorded assessment of need and objectives of intervention.

3.3.5 Accurate, legible, factual, contemporaneous and attributed records and reports of occupational therapy intervention shall be kept in order to provide information for colleagues and legal purposes such as client access and court reports.

Regular audit of the standard of note keeping and documentation will help in ensuring the department's standards are being maintained.

CONFLICT

Conflict is most likely to arise when the client and/or carers, or even other team members, perceive that the service provided by the occupational therapist is not meeting their expectations. Occupational therapists must, therefore, clearly identify the aims and objectives of their treatment plan and intervention while also realizing that they may be the focus of anger if the whole situation is becoming frustrating and unsatisfactory. This can easily occur when dealing with tragic circumstances in which someone has a life-threatening illness with a disability, and the focus of hopelessness is transferred to the occupational therapist regarding tangible pieces of equipment.

For example, on a pre-discharge home assessment, the occupational therapist takes the client from the hospital to the home for a needs assessment, visits the home with the client from hospital. The client's wife is angry and specifically requests an item of equipment and focuses on this, strongly declining other help that the occupational therapist or other healthcare professionals feel would be of use. Once that item of equipment is provided, another problem arises and the occupational therapist becomes the focus of this problem. The basic problem is unresolved anger and denial at the diagnosis and the occupational therapist simply happens to be in the line of fire. The multiprofessional team, therefore, needs a consistent approach so as not to be sidetracked and to ensure the real issues are addressed.

Conflict can be an energizing and vitalizing force if properly managed. It can have both positive and negative outcomes as it allows expression of worries and concerns and creates an opportunity for problems to be resolved. It has to be accepted that conflict is an inevitable feature of life in complex organizations and may occur at personal, interpersonal and group levels. If handled correctly, it can be contained and channelled positively. Ways in which conflict can be resolved include compromise, in which the parties involved decide on a solution of give and take, solve the underlying problem or avoid it altogether.

Conflict can be linked to aggression, which can take the form of disagreement, anger, verbal abuse or violence. Different interventions are needed for diffusing and handling aggression as particular situations arise. Often, the client or carers need the opportunity to express their feelings – they need to be allowed to be angry in a safe environment, and it is important to listen to them rather than shout them down. An empathetic approach will often help to diffuse the situation, not by identifying with them ('I know how you feel') but by acknowledging that it is understandable that they are angry and talking through the situation.

Aggression is a means of gaining power over others. Clients and carers are in the position of having lost control over their lives because of the disease and impairment and so they need to have some autonomy over decisions. A client may not want a whole string of different healthcare professionals coming in and out of his or her house. Compromise is, therefore, necessary in order to maintain the client safely without taking over.

Occupational therapists might consider whom they work with and against in their work setting. For example, an occupational therapist might work well with clients, carers and multiprofessional staff but might come into conflict with budget holders over the provision of service. Once this has been identified, it might facilitate some resolution.

Suppose the occupational therapist visits a young client with a life-threatening illness, and the mother will not let the occupational therapist talk to the client but instead berates the entire service and tells the occupational therapist what is needed. The occupational therapist needs to consider:

- confidentiality – how much the mother knows;
- boundary-setting, making clear the occupational therapist's role;
- allowing the mother to express concerns and anger and acknowledging these issues;
- addressing the issues;
- asking the mother what she wants for her child;
- explaining that the occupational therapist is ultimately working for the client;
- giving back control to the family and facilitating a situation where they work together to accept the multiprofessional team and service's input.

Lanciotti and Hopkins (1995) describe proactive principles when dealing with hostility in Appendix 4. Reflection following a case of conflict can be carried out in formal supervision or using informal support.

LOSS

Loss can take many forms: it can involve loss of a job, aspirations, home, security, children, a partner (in death or divorce), of a body part or loss of self-esteem, independence, friends, health or time. Losses are multifaceted; loss of mobility alone can lead to changes in:

- role
- physical integrity
- mental integrity
- independence
- dignity
- faith
- life expectancy
- autonomy
- comfort, privacy
- social relationships, work
- body image
- weight changes
- unfamiliar emotions and behaviour
- self-esteem
- sexual function
- bodily function
- hopes
- freedom
- dreams
- quality of life.

Most healthcare professionals are likely to be the focus of the client's feelings of loss at one time or another. Occupational therapists typically find that they are blamed when there is a delay in the provision of equipment. Equipment is a tangible item on which people can focus their feelings of loss. There is a danger here of transference of hopelessness from the client, carer or colleagues to the therapist. Occupational therapists need to be aware of this but they should be able to recognize their own feelings and those of the client.

Having said this, non-provision of equipment can lead to delayed discharge from hospital. It is a vital part of the occupational therapy programme to anticipate problems and not end up mopping up a crisis. With increased demand for resources and decreased funding, occupational therapists need to be aware of this potential cause of stress.

GRIEF

Although there are observable and well-documented patterns of grief, there is no such thing as a 'normal time span for grief'. This can be very distressing and even annoying to relatives and friends who may think that 'it is time he got over it'. The grieving process could well commence prior to death. The client and carers may grieve for loss of function (mobility, body image and role) as well as loss of life.

Grief is a normal psychological response to any significant loss and there is no correct reaction for healthcare professionals. It depends on the individual. Occupational therapists can play a role in supporting the client, carers and each other by helping them adjust to loss in their own way. Table 2.1 shows the stages that people may go through.

Occupational therapists have counselling skills and techniques that are used within this area of work. However, within most units there will be other members of the multiprofessional team who are employed as counsellors and they have more extensive training in this field. Occupational therapists can use their skills to recognize the need for referral to other agencies when this feel appropriate. Simple techniques can be used to build rapport with clients and to encourage them to express themselves more openly so that the occupational therapist can assess whether counselling is necessary. These may include avoiding closed questions, i.e. questions that can be answered monosyllabically with 'yes' or 'no'. This can be done by using words like 'what, where, when, why, who'. For example, the question 'Did the doctor tell you about your illness?' can be changed to 'What or how much did the doctor tell you about your illness?'

Reflection, which involves mirroring and repeating key points of conversation to clarify them, encourages the client to continue speaking. For example, a middle-aged man recovering from an amputation says, 'I'll never get used to this. Sometimes I think I would be better off if I'd died. What's the point of living when you are a cripple?' The response might be 'So you feel you'll never get used to your amputation, that you sometimes think you'd have been better off dying, and you wonder what the point of living is?' Mirroring, reflecting and clarifying enables the occupational therapist to check that he or she has understood clients' words correctly before encouraging them to share their concerns.

CULTURAL ISSUES

Cooper (1997) advises that healthcare professionals should acquire background knowledge about how disease is viewed within specific communities and about what determines people's individuality and status within various cultural hierarchies. Our society is multicultural yet there remains the need for greater understanding of the variety of ethnic and religious groups that make up our communities. This does not exclude occupational therapists from holding their own religious beliefs but reinforces the need to understand and respect the needs and requirements of the client.

Assumptions must never be made about how devout an individual is regarding their faith or culture, nor about how the dynamics and support of the client's family and carers will be influenced by religion or culture. The occupational therapist should establish whether the client holds strong

Table 2.1 'Normal' patterns of bereavement behaviour

	Denial Death of spouse up to 2 weeks	Developing Awareness 2 weeks–2 years	Resolution 2 years–5 years
Physical reaction	Shock	Loss of vitality. Physical symptoms of stress. Irrational behaviour often coming in waves lasting 20–60 minutes Psychosomatic illness, often parallels symptoms of deceased (may not be reversed)	
Emotional	Numbness Cottonwool feeling Denial	Outbursts of grief (pining, crying, exhaustion) Depression or sadness Anger – against deceased, medicine, God ('why?') Loss of confidence and self-approval Guilt ('if only') Loneliness – especially in older bereaved	The resolve that one will cope; Sense of detachment allowing freedom of action; Feeling it is now OK to enjoy social contacts, etc.
External factors affecting behaviour	Circumstances of death and funeral arrangements Family Religious beliefs and culture	Idealizing of the deceased Financial loss or gain Loss of status Anniversaries Society's disapproval of overt emotions and avoidance of death	Acceptance of new status by society; Role of bereavement organizations.

(From *Letting Go*, Ainsworth-Smith and Speck (1982) cited in Cooper (1997)) religious beliefs that will impact upon treatment programmes. There may be relevant issues regarding food restrictions, dress code and prohibition of participation in dressing practice. The occupational therapist needs to find out what the patient will and will not do, both in a domestic setting and in treatment sessions. The family or religious adviser might also be able to advise about what the client is able to do. Difficulties are unlikely to arise if one is honest and says, 'you tell me what is and is not permitted,' and if one shows genuine respect and interest in the client's culture.

Illness might affect how clients' communities view and accept them. Within certain cultural groups, body-image alteration and dysfunction can affect an individual's standing within the family, the community, at work and within the religious community. It could even lead to exclusion from worship in a holy place. Specific difficulties arise with hair loss, amputation of body parts and stomas.

HAIR LOSS

Hair loss is common among western males and is associated with the ageing process. For women it is perceived as far more damaging and is a clear indication to others of a serious illness. Although there are wigs, turbans or scarves available, and these can be acceptable to some, hair loss can be emotionally devastating as styling, colour and length make social statements about the individual.

Other societies place far greater emphasis on hair and hair loss. Amongst some Cantonese-speaking communities, hair is a symbol of power to absorb life forces and a medium for losing toxins and impurities that arise from disease and from the death of a family member. Hair loss leads to fears regarding an individual's ability to recover from illness.

The Sikh faith views the intactness of the body as extremely important and hair loss diminishes both men and women. In African cultures hair loss can be an outward sign of loss of fertility. Rastafarians, in particular, see dreadlocks as symbols of black dignity and inward power, so loss of hair may be devastating to their self-image. Orthodox Jewish women customarily have short hair or a shorn head whereas other Jewish women value their hair. The more strict Christian faiths such as the Amish, the Taylorites and the Exclusive Brethren wear their hair long as a sign of God's favour.

BREAST LOSS DUE TO MASTECTOMY

As well as feelings of loss of sexuality, there may be shame associated with loss of a breast due to feelings of a lack of self-worth influenced by culture and religion. Western society values the breast shape and size. Altered body shape certainly affects women's feelings of self-confidence and how others view them.

STOMAS

Colostomies, ileostomies and urostomies may not only threaten the individual's self-esteem and body image but may also alter their ability to worship. This can lead to ostracism and may be viewed as uncleanliness. The Islamic faith does not allow ablutions during prayer and, as stomas cannot be controlled voluntarily, an individual may need to leave and start prayers again after each wash. Occupational therapists should be aware of the implications of cultural issues on such fundamental tasks.

SPIRITUALITY

Law *et al.* (1997) discuss how spirituality is the manifestation of a higher self, a spiritual direction or greater purpose which nurtures people through life events and choices. How a person chooses to envision this guiding principle depends upon how they evolve as individuals. Heminiak (1996) defined spirituality as being viewed as a way of living that demonstrates essential values regarding the role of the individual in the world. For some, spirituality is a religious vision, for others it is much less clear, being purely a feeling or sense of meaning. The Occupational Performance process comprises information gathering, assessing, establishing the treatment plan, carrying out treatment and evaluation. Spirituality should be reflected in the whole process and is integral to every step, is not just a performance component but is a central feature of the person (Rose, 1999). The client has to be the focus of the process so that there is ownership. While the client guides the process, the occupational therapist reflects the client's values, beliefs and preferences in the treatment programme that they help to establish.

Spirituality is at the heart of assessing which occupations are meaningful to clients and in building meaningful occupation into targeted outcomes, action plans and implementation. It is a fundamental, central part of the process of enabling self-determination, relating services to life experiences and making occupation meaningful (Stanton *et al.*, 1997).

Law *et al.* (1997) describe spirituality as being an innate essence of self, a quality of being uniquely and truly human, an expression of will, drive and motivation, a source of self-determination and personal control and a guide for expressing choice. Because people are spiritual beings, they should be treated as unique. Their values, beliefs and goals are, therefore, essential to their spirituality. When occupations are used therapeutically, they must have relevance and meaning for each client and have clear therapeutic aims and objectives and also be of that client's choice. Appendix 5 shows the therapeutic effects of facilitating self-expression (Stoter 1996).

When clients face difficult times such as dealing with the diagnosis and treatment of a life-threatening disease, they are likely to take on different values and beliefs; occupational therapists must reflect with people on occupations that hold significance for them. Unruh *et al.* (1999) describe how meanings attributed to various occupations and the environments in which they occur may influence the degree to which an occupation contributes to spiritual well-being. They discuss how the professional literature suggests that we have a spiritual drive that compels us to seek purpose and meaning from life and, through our occupations, we address our own unique spiritual needs. They conclude that enabling spiritual well-being through occupation is an important concern for occupational therapists particularly for clients who are facing a significant health threat.

SUMMARY

This chapter has identified potential areas of stress and burnout which the occupational therapist needs to address in order to perform effectively in the clinical areas of oncology and palliative care. Support mechanisms must be developed to facilitate good working practice and ensure the patient is receiving the best possible care.

ACTION POINTS

1. Establish a concise, clear, professional explanation of the occupational therapist's role to present to colleagues within the multiprofessional team.
2. Discuss coping mechanisms for occupational therapists when working with a client group with life-threatening illnesses. How is this incorporated in clinical practice?
3. Identify training needs when working in this clinical area and how these can be implemented.

REFERENCES

Bennett, S. (1991) Issues confronting occupational therapists working with terminally ill patients. *British Journal of Occupational Therapy*, **54**(1), 8–10.
Brewin, T. B. (1991) Three ways of giving bad news. *Lancet*, **337**(8751), 1207–9.
Bye, R. A. (1998) When clients are dying: Occupational therapists' perspectives. *The Occupational Therapy Journal of Research*, **18**(1), 3–24.
College of Occupational Therapists (2005) *Code of Ethics and Professional Conduct. Occupation matters*, COT, London.
Cooper, J. (1997) *Occupational Therapy in Oncology & Palliative Care*, Whurr, London.
Cooper, J. and Littlechild, B. (2004) A study of occupational therapy interventions in oncology and palliative care. *International Journal of Therapy and Rehabilitation*, **11**(7), 329–33.

Coulter, A., Entwistle, V. and Gilbert, D. (1999) Sharing decisions with patients: Is the information good enough? *British Medical Journal*, **3**(18), 318–22.

Department of Health (2000) *The NHS Cancer Plan. A plan for investment. A plan for reform*, HMSO, London.

Faulkner, A. and Maguire, P. (1994) *Talking to Cancer Patients and their Relatives*, Oxford Medical Publications, Oxford.

Gamage, S. L., McMahon, P. S. and Shanahan, P. M. (1976) The occupational therapist and terminal illness. Learning to cope with death. *American Journal of Occupational Therapy*, **30**(5), 294–9.

Glass, E. and Cluxton, D. (2004) Truth-telling: Ethical issues in clinical practice. *Journal of Hospice and Palliative Nursing*, **6**(4), 232–43.

Heminiak, D. A. (1996) *The Core of Human Spirituality*, State University of New York, Albany, NY.

Kaye, P. (1994) *Breaking Bad News*, EPL Publications, Northampton.

Lanciotti, L. and Hopkins, A. (1995) Breaking the cycle. *Nursing Standard*, **10**(11), 22–4.

Law, M., Baptiste, S. and Mills, J. (1995) Client-centred practice: What does it mean and does it make a difference? *Canadian Journal of Occupational Therapy*, **62**(5), 250–6.

Law, M., Polatojko, H., Baptiste, S. and Townsend, S. (1997) Core concepts of occupational therapy, in *Enabling Occupation: An occupational therapy perspective* (ed. E. Townsend), CAOT, Ontario.

Mead, N. and Bower, P. (2000) Patient-centredness: A conceptual framework and review of the empirical literature. *Soc Sci Med*, **51**(7), 1087–110.

NHS Executive (2000) *Cancer Information Strategy*, HMSO, London.

Rose, A. (1999) Spirituality and palliative care: The attitudes of occupational therapists. *British Journal of Occupational Therapy*, **62**(7), 307–12.

Royal Society of Medicine (2000) Effective health care: Informing, communicating and sharing decisions with people who have cancer. *Royal Society of Medicine Bulletin*, **6**(6), 1–8.

Smith, C. (2000) The role of health professionals in informing cancer patients: Findings from the teamwork project (phase one). *Health Expectations*, **3**(3), 217–19.

Stanton, S., Thompson-Franson, T. and Kramer, C. (1997) Linking concepts to a process for working with clients, in *Enabling Occupation: An occupational therapy perspective* (ed. E. Townsend), CAOT, Ontario.

Stoter, D. (1996) Spiritual care, in *Palliative Care for People with Cancer* (eds J. Penson and R. Fisher), Edward Arnold, London.

Unruh, A. M., Smith, N. and Scammell, C. (1999) The occupation of gardening in life-threatening illness: A qualitative pilot project, *Canadian Journal of Occupational Therapy*, **67**(1), 70–7.

Watterson, J., Lowrie, D., Vockins, H., Ewer-Smith, C. and Cooper, J. (2004) Rehabilitation goals identified by inpatients with cancer using the COPM, *International Journal of Therapy and Rehabilitation*, **11**(5), 219–25.

3 Occupational Therapy Approach in Symptom Control

JILL COOPER

Ingham and Portenoy (2004) describe how, for patients, the disease experience is inextricably linked to symptoms and the resultant distress. They suggest that symptoms are inherently subjective and that they are perceptions, usually conveyed by language. Occupational therapists use a problem-solving approach in addressing symptoms and dysfunctions – physical, emotional, psychological and psychosocial.

Occupational therapists make a valuable contribution in alleviating certain symptoms, the intervention being symptom-led rather than disease- or diagnosis-led. Because occupational therapy is concerned with the functional implications of symptoms, the occupational therapist also tries to plan ahead and anticipate functional problems rather than waiting for a crisis to occur.

Clipp and George (1992) reported on a study, the results of which showed that patients' subjective reporting disagreed with some of the objective assessments carried out by healthcare professionals. The optimal approach must, therefore, be to include the patient's perspective of symptoms as well as objective clinical assessments. It must also be noted that standardized, validated assessments can be very tiring for the patient when they are administered. Great care and expertise are required, therefore, in selecting appropriate assessments so that the patient's well-being is not compromised by the assessment itself.

Symptoms are multifaceted and multidimensional and as many as seven symptoms may be present at any one time in advanced disease (Dunlop, 1989). Symptoms also usually change, either remitting or recurring. This reinforces the necessity to have assessment measures that are simple and brief enough to limit patient burden and encourage compliance (Ingham *et al.*, 1996). It also reinforces the need to have continuous review to ensure the occupational therapist is working towards the priorities of the individual, and that priorities are still realistic and achievable.

Occupational Therapy in Oncology and Palliative Care. Edited by J. Cooper
© 2006 John Wiley & Sons Ltd

The occupational therapist's role in management of symptoms is to:

- maintain up-to-date professional knowledge of the symptom and its treatments;
- explore the meaning of the symptom to the individual;
- explore the impact of the symptom on individuals and their family or carers;
- investigate how it stops them from carrying out their required objectives in life.

The 12 common symptoms treated in palliative care are:

weakness 82%	swollen legs 46%
dry mouth 68%	nausea 42%
anorexia 58%	constipation 36%
depression 52%	vomiting 32%
pain 46%	confusion 30%
insomnia 46%	dyspnoea 30%

(Dunlop, 1989)

PROBLEM-SOLVING APPROACH

Cooper (1997) describes how the occupational therapy intervention takes a problem-solving approach to symptom control. Problem solving forms the basis for analysing the client's needs and enabling the client to cope with dysfunction. Illness creates physical, psychological, emotional, social and financial problems. Even though a client's situation can appear overwhelming, the occupational therapist will find it helpful to identify specific problems and to try to resolve them.

In all occupational therapy treatment plans, the first step is to establish rapport and to set baseline aims and objectives. The problem-solving strategy can then be set out, for example:

- trying to identify the underlying difficulty;
- establishing and discussing the particular event that might contribute to the initiation of the problem;
- setting achievable aims to deal with that event by breaking the problem down into stages;
- discussing techniques and methods to cope with these stages;
- discussing the possible outcome to the successful problem-solving strategy and what to do next;
- making it clear that the strategy might not always succeed but that it is necessary to persevere.

This facilitates patients in applying the coping strategy themselves and taking control.

As stated above, many patients with advanced disease experience a range of symptoms, often simultaneously. Although symptoms are described in isolation in this chapter, they are seldom seen as the only presenting symptom in the clinical setting.

Pushpangadan and Burns (1996) stated that the community occupational therapist has an important role in relation to the provision of equipment, adaptations and advice regarding home care, and the need for skilled assessment. In addition to addressing the physical help available to support patients and their families, there are other considerations including intellectual, emotional and psychosocial needs. A consensus of occupational therapists specializing in oncology and palliative care, Occupational Therapy Specialist Section in HIV/AIDS, Oncology and Palliative Care Education (HOPE), produced a book in conjunction with the College of Occupational Therapists (HOPE, 2004) in which occupational therapy interventions were highlighted in symptom management. It discusses three specific themes of special relevance on which occupational therapy focuses:

LIFESTYLE MANAGEMENT

The occupational therapist can:

- work with people with cancer and family/carers to achieve balance in life;
- help them assess what priorities are most important to them – including social and spiritual priorities;
- help them find occupation which is meaningful to them;
- take into account the influences of culture;
- provide a crucial link between care in hospital and living at home.

FATIGUE MANAGEMENT

The occupational therapist can:

- recognize that fatigue affects people's ability to function and be independent;
- provide information and advice to people with cancer and family/carers about strategies to manage their fatigue and conserve energy;
- help them understand the need to adjust to change and accept some dependency and fluctuation;
- help them establish realistic expectations and goals;
- use reduced energy levels as an opportunity for people to establish what is important to them, and what their priorities should be;
- help them adapt their lifestyle to meet their changed energy levels, providing equipment and adapting the environment where necessary.

SELF-ESTEEM

The occupational therapist can:

- recognize that a person's inner feeling of self-worth influences their motivation;
- recognize that involvement in purposeful activity affects feelings of self-worth;
- help people explore their feelings, recognize who they are and what is important to them;
- help people acknowledge their values, and their role within their family and the community;
- help them adapt to these changing roles;
- help them reflect on their current and past achievements to underpin self-worth.

Reproduced by kind permission of HOPE and COT

Three key areas of intervention in which occupational therapists are specializing are:

- fatigue management including weakness;
- breathlessness management;
- relaxation and anxiety management including depression.

These are explored in greater depths in the following chapters. Interventions into other symptoms are summarized below.

FEEDING PROBLEMS, INCLUDING DRY MOUTH
AND ANOREXIA

When the patient complains of a dry mouth, the nursing intervention is vital to address this uncomfortable and distressing symptom. Oral hygiene is essential with particular attention to dental care and dentures. Oral infections, ill-fitting teeth, medication and ulcers also result in rapid weight loss.

Other issues involving feeding difficulties not only have physical implications for the patient, but are distressing for the family, as most cultures place great importance on the individual's appetite and weight. Cooper (1997) describes how feeding is such a basic aspect of daily living that any problems must be investigated. There may be underlying difficulties of nausea and vomiting, lack of appetite (anorexia) and altered taste sensation, in which cases the dietitian must assess these.

Cognitive dysfunction is likely to affect hand–eye coordination, in which case help of one person is needed particularly if adapted cutlery is ineffective.

If the patient is at home, issues of meal preparation and carrying it to the eating area need addressing. Feeding problems can give rise to psychological difficulties. Energy, or calorie, intake and mood are directly related so reduction in food intake can cause negative changes in mood. Clients who are unable to eat well may feel guilty because they are not eating and this in turn upsets their carers.

Cooper (1997) advises strategies to support dietetic advice as the occupational therapist is likely to be more involved in ongoing treatment sessions:

- giving smaller portions of food but increasing the frequency of these smaller meals;
- establishing which foods the patients can chew and swallow without effort;
- encouraging eating whenever and whatever the patient wants rather than worrying about set meal times, particularly as appetite often reduces later in the day;
- indulging cravings in order to increase calorie intake, although a compromise may be needed if excessive amounts of particular foods cause dietetic concern, including alcohol;
- providing feeding aids as necessary to help with grip, management of tremors and limited range of movement.

In addition, the occupational therapist can assist in body image issues (Shearsmith-Farthing, 2001), and pressure care intervention as necessary (Cooper, 1997).

PAIN

Pain is a well documented symptom, with pharmacological intervention clearly prescribed in the medical clinical setting. Cooper (1997) discusses how occupational therapists work in pain control clinics with chronic pain syndromes, but the oncology and palliative care setting are a quite separate clinical entity. The palliative care team aims for optimum pain control or relief: pain does not have the same behavioural or cognitive element as chronic pain control.

Foley (2004) describes the multidimensional aspects of pain in both cancer-related acute pain and cancer-related chronic pain syndromes. Acute pain is most likely to be associated with diagnostic and treatment interventions, for example, biopsies, chemotherapy and radiotherapy (Cherny and Portenoy, 1994). The chronic pain with which the occupational therapist is likely to become involved in advanced stage disease may be due to:

- multiple bony metastases in any part of the skeletal system;
- visceral pain from tumour infiltration in the internal organs;

- neuropathic pain from tumour infiltration to nervous system;
- post-chemotherapy, post-radiotherapy or post-surgical pain.

Although the main treatment for pain is pharmacological, the occupational therapist helps identify the impact that pain has on the individual and address emotional issues by:

- establishing the effects of the pain on the individuals' ability to function as they would choose to do so;
- establishing how it affects the patients' whole family dynamics, their role and capacity to lead a productive life even within the constraints of the changes caused by the pain;
- setting goals and priorities with the patients, which are reviewed regularly and adjusted as necessary;
- working with individuals using occupational therapy core skills and interventions to facilitate improved quality of life, assessing lifestyle management, energy conservation, anxiety management and ergonomics;
- assessing for and prescribing equipment to aid independence and comfort.

Lloyd and Coggles (1988) state that successful pain management can be achieved through coordinated efforts of the team members of the cancer care team. Occupational therapy is vital to the pain management service and can help modify perceptions of pain and individuals' lifestyles.

INSOMNIA

Sateia and Santulli (2004) define insomnia as a subjective complaint of poor sleep by patients. They describe common causes of insomnia in advanced disease as being depression, anxiety, cognitive impairment/disorder, pain, nausea and vomiting, respiratory distress, medications, disruption of normal routine and restless leg syndrome or periodic limb movement. It can be very distressing and exacerbate fatigue which they may also be experiencing.

The impact on the carers can be that their sleep is also disturbed so the whole family unit may have altered sleep patterns and fatigue. As well as teaching relaxation techniques, the occupational therapist can explore different options for posture and positioning in bed, and techniques and equipment to enable safe bed mobility and transfers. As with all the symptoms, it is important to acknowledge the impact of poor sleep on the patient and family. If insomnia is creating a major problem in their quality of life, the fact that the team is recognizing and addressing it can be of great reassurance to them.

SWOLLEN LEGS, INCLUDING LYMPHOEDEMA

Swollen limbs result in a range of difficulties for patients including pain, altered body image, excessive sweating, discomfort and mobility and transfer problems. Lymphoedema is tissue swelling due to a failure of lymph drainage and may be congenital or the result of obliteration or obstruction of lymph channels (Badger, 1987).

If the swelling is due to lymphoedema, this should be addressed by the specialist lymphoedema therapist in the specific clinic where a course of pressure bandaging is provided followed by compression hosiery to maintain the limb volume. The compression hosiery can be difficult to tolerate and the patient may have resulting loss of function and dexterity.

Functional implications are difficulties with:

- everyday activities such as washing and dressing;
- flexibility;
- balance which affects safety in transfers into/out of bath or shower;
- exercise tolerance.

The occupational therapist can assist with:

- assessing mobility, transfers and self-care activities with a view to teaching alternative techniques of coping and prescribing equipment to aid independence;
- providing splints to enable comfort and correct joint positioning particularly for upper limb lymphoedema;
- providing advice on energy conservation and safety issues;
- assessing for and prescribing equipment, e.g. wheelchair, armchair, hoist to ensure transfers and mobility are safe and that skin integrity is not compromised, for example, large equipment that will not rub the fragile, swollen skin.

NAUSEA AND VOMITING

Nausea and vomiting are very unpleasant symptoms that are reported as highly distressing to patients, particularly those undergoing chemotherapy regimes (Meuser *et al.*, 2001). They may be caused by a variety of reasons including drugs, anxiety, brain metastases, oral thrush, gastric irritation, squashed stomach syndrome, gastric outflow obstruction, constipation or cough.

Anti-emetics are the first line of treatment in addressing nausea and vomiting, and occupational therapy intervention has developed relaxation and breathing techniques to help alleviate the tension and apprehension which is likely to occur with this symptom. In addition to this approach, HOPE (2004) states that occupational therapy can:

- address the difficulties of meal/drink preparation and explore alternatives such as using ready meals to avoid tiring cooking sessions or smells which may exacerbate this symptom;
- liaise with other team members to achieve a comfortable position for dependent patients with dysphagia;
- liaise with other team members about oral hygiene, and how to cope with extra laundry and general hygiene that result from episodes of vomiting;
- provide support, advice and education for the family and carers on coping with this symptom and emphasize the psychological as well as physical implications.

CONSTIPATION, DIARRHOEA AND URINARY PROBLEMS

The adverse effects of medication and disease progression can include these symptoms which make the patient's life miserable and undignified. These symptoms can be painful and tiring and require immediate medical assessment. The occupational therapist can contribute to their management by addressing:

- actual access to the toilet and bathroom. If the patient is very weak, there may be mobility needs or there might be the need for strategically placed handrails and equipment to ensure transfers onto/off the toilet and into/out shower and bath are safe;
- the need for adapting clothing to make it easier to get on and off;
- the liaison with the multiprofessional team regarding maintenance of hygiene and obtaining help for laundry as well as financial support for the extra care and washing required.

CONFUSION

Confusion is the most common and serious neuropsychiatric complication of advanced disease, prevalence ranging from 25–85% in the last weeks of life (Fainsinger and Young, 1991).

Causes may be:

- direct central nervous system metastases;
- side-effects from treatment such as medication toxicity, chemotherapy and radiotherapy;

- infection, such as urinary tract or kidney;
- disease process resulting in hypercalcaemia and other chemical imbalances.

The implications are very distressing for the family and carers, and frightening and disorientating for the individual themselves. The occupational therapist's role is to:

- assist in the thorough assessment including cognitive and functional assessment;
- establish whether the patient can cope safely with help;
- work with the patient, family and multiprofessional team to ensure the safest solution to support all those involved in the patient's care.

RADIATION-INDUCED BRACHIAL PLEXOPATHY (RIBP)

Radiation-induced brachial plexopathy is damage caused to the nerves and tissues adjacent to the clavicle and under the armpit due to treatment with ionizing radiation for treatment of breast cancer (Cooper, 1998). This side-effect is seen very rarely but can lead to irreversible symptoms as fibrous tissue constricts the brachial plexus, ranging from lymphoedema, hypersensitivity, lack of sensation, muscle wasting or a combination of these. The occupational therapist forms part of the multiprofessional approach to these distressing symptoms which may present in some cases 7–10 years after the radiotherapy finishes. The occupational therapist's role is:

- to establish rapport to identify areas of dysfunction;
- to devise strategies to compensate for dysfunction with assessment for and provision of equipment to enable independence;
- to assess for most appropriate intervention from splinting to compensation techniques;
- to regular review to provide continuity of care and regular evaluation of symptoms;
- to provide psychological and emotional support with relaxation training and anxiety and fatigue management.

SPINAL CORD COMPRESSION

Spinal cord compression can be of sudden onset and, consequently, be a huge shock for clients and their carers. In addition to dealing with the physical implications, the psychological adjustment is enormous for them and the occupational therapist needs to help them in adjusting to the disability. As this can be at a time of advanced disease, there might not be enough time for psychological adjustment and the multiprofessional team needs to be aware of the very high level of support required by all those involved.

Spinal cord compression is compression of the thecal sac by a tumour in the epidural space, either at the level of the spinal cord or cauda equina, compressing the spinal canal. Malignant tumours may be classified as primary, i.e. arising from the tissue in the spinal cord or spinal canal, or secondary, i.e. arising as metastatic solid tumours. Eva and Lord (2003) state that malignant spinal cord compression occurs in up to 5% of all patients with systemic cancer.

Clinical features depend on the extent and rate of the disease progression. Motor symptoms vary from initially including fatigue, gait disturbance, and back pain to change in urinary and sphincter control. Cervical spine disease results in quadriplegia, thoracic spine disease in paraplegia, lumbar disease disease affects L4, L5 and sacral nerve roots. Sensory symptoms include sensory loss or paraesthesia, alteration in light touch, proprioception and joint position sense, and tendon reflexes are often affected.

Acute cord compression is a surgical emergency in order to decompress the obstruction. Cortico-steroids are prescribed initially until more definite treatment such as surgical decompression can be instituted. This is advocated to:

- establish the diagnosis;
- treat a single site of suspected involvement;
- treat progression despite radiation therapy;
- treat vertebral instability, collapse with bone impinging on the spinal cord or displacement

(Loblaw and Laperierre, 1998)

Surgery is not advocated for metastases from prostate or breast cancer, myeloma and lymphoma, which are likely (70–88%) to respond to radiotherapy (Abrahm, 1999). Radiotherapy may be given but there is a finite dosage that can be given, so if the spinal cord compression recurs, this may not be possible. CancerSource.com (2005) recommends that, while it is not possible to prevent spinal cord compression, it is possible to prevent it from getting worse. Symptoms must be addressed urgently.

Occupational therapy intervention requires a holistic approach as the impact on the patient's and family's lives is enormous. The multiprofessional team aims ultimately for optimum functional independence but needs to be flexible as the prognosis can be poor. Each service should have a clear protocol for the management of spinal cord compression to enable staff in their treatment of this condition. Cooper (1997) describes the stages of onset and functional implications:

Early stages may include localized back pain. Radicular pain limits functional activities such as bending down to put on shoes and clothes, standing during activities and walking. Psychological effects of pain may include depression, fear of mobilizing, tension, lack of sleep and anxiety, which result in lethargy and fatigue. Occupational therapy intervention comprises advising and teaching alternative methods to carry out tasks to minimize pain and discomfort. Anxiety management may be appropriate to enable patients to cope with their feelings as well as to assist them in understanding the condition and to adapt to the change in functional independence. A regular treatment programme is required to restore confidence and self-esteem. Issues relating to employment and driving may still be relevant, with individual circumstances being assessed and addressed depending on the level of function.

Advanced stages may range from leg weakness, loss of muscle power, atrophy, foot-drop, reduced balance, ataxia, reduced coordination and muscle spasm to include paraesthesia or paraplegia and may still be painful. Occupational therapy intervention comprises assessment of mobility and transfers, close liaison with the physiotherapist as well as with all of the multiprofessional team, and, depending on the individual's dysfunction, wheelchair and pressure care provision. If aiming for sliding transfers, the wheelchair and commode will require removable arms, though hoisting may be preferable if the skin is broken on the sacrum and/or buttocks. Even though patients may be young, it must not be presumed that they are as strong as young fit people with paraplegia, as they have advanced disease and their arms may not be strong enough to enable them to transfer independently. Prompt provision of all appropriate equipment to enable optimum functional independence at home is required as the prognosis may be limited.

SUMMARY

The problem-solving approach in occupational therapy does not provide a set answer for an individual's approach. When an occupational therapist is faced with a client with spinal cord compression, for example, there is no checklist to tick off to tell them what to do. It may be necessary to:

- reflect on the issues discussed in Chapter 2;
- be aware of the background of the disease – not only the diagnosis, but also the treatment;
- appreciate issues the client and carers are facing;
- use core psychological and physical occupational therapy skills.

When selecting the appropriate occupational therapy intervention, the therapeutic aims and benefits to the client are the main consideration.

ACTION POINTS

1. Explore the psychological and physical implications of any of the main symptoms and how occupational therapy might address these.
2. Explore the support required for the occupational therapist and other members of the multiprofessional team, including professional training in the conditions as well as personal needs.
3. Carry out a literature review of specific symptoms and critically evaluate the occupational therapy role involved.

REFERENCES

Abrahm, J. L. (1999) Management of pain and spinal cord compression in patients with advanced cancer. *Annals of Internal Medicine*, **131**(1), 37–46.

Badger, C. (1987) Lymphoedema: Management of patients with advanced cancer. *Professional Nurse*, **2**(4), 100–2.

CancerSource.com (2005) Spinal Cord Compression: www.cancersource.com accessed July 2005.

Cherny, N. and Portenoy, R. K. (1994) Cancer pain: Principles of assessment and syndromes, in *Textbook of Pain* (eds P. D. Wall and R. Melzack), Churchill Livingstone, Edinburgh.

Clipp, E. C. and George, L. K. (1992) Patients with cancer and their spouse caregivers. Perceptions of the illness experience. *Cancer*, **69**(4), 1074–9.

Cooper, J. (1997) *Occupational Therapy in Oncology and Palliative Care*, Whurr, London.

Cooper, J. (1998) Occupational therapy intervention with radiation-induced brachial plexopathy. *European Journal of Cancer Care*, **7**(2), 88–92.

Dunlop, G. M. (1989) A study of the relative frequency and importance of gastrointestinal symptoms and weakness in patients with far advanced cancer. *Palliative Medicine*, **4**(1), 37–43.

Eva, G. and Lord, S. (2003) Rehabilitation in malignant spinal cord compression. *European Journal of Palliative Care*, **10**(4), 148–50.

Fainsinger, R. and Young, C. (1991) Cognitive failure in a terminally ill patient. *Journal of Pain and Symptom Management*, **6**(8), 492–4.

Foley, K. (2004) Acute and chronic cancer pain syndromes, in *Oxford Textbook of Palliative Medicine,* 3rd edn (eds D. Doyle, G. Hanks, N. Cherny and K. Calman), Oxford University Press, Oxford.

HOPE (HIV/AIDS, Oncology and Palliative Care Education) (2004) *Occupational Therapy Intervention in Cancer: Guidance for professionals, managers and decision-makers,* College of Occupational Therapists, London.

Ingham, J. M. and Portenoy, R. K. (2004) Patient evaluation and outcome measures, in *Oxford Textbook of Palliative Medicine,* 3rd edn (eds D. Doyle, G. Hanks, N. Cherny and K. Calman), Oxford University Press, Oxford.

Ingham, J. M., Siedman, A., Yao, T. J., Lepore, J. and Portenoy, R. (1996) An exploratory study of frequent pain measurement in a cancer clinical trial. *Quality of Life*

Research: An International Journal of Quality of Life Aspects of Treatment, Care and Rehabilitation, **5**(5), 503–7.

Lloyd, C. and Coggles, L. (1988) Contribution of occupational therapy to pain management in cancer patients with metastatic breast disease. *American Journal of Hospice Care*, **5**(6), 36–8.

Loblaw, D. A. and Laperierre, N. J. (1998) Emergency treatment of malignant extradural spinal cord compression: An evidence-based guideline. *Journal of Clinical Oncology*, **16**(4), 1613–24.

Meuser, T., Pietruck, C., Radbruch, L., Stute, P., Lehmann, K. A. and Grond, S. (2001) Symptoms during cancer pain treatment following WHO guidelines: A longitudinal follow-up study of symptoms, prevalence, severity and etiology. *Pain*, **93**(3), 247–57.

Pushpangadan, M. and Burns, E. (1996) Caring for older people: Community services: Health. *British Medical Journal*, **313**(7060), 805–8.

Sateia, M. J. and Santulli, R. B. (2004) Sleep in palliative care. *Oxford Textbook of Palliative Medicine*, 3rd edn (eds D. Doyle, G. Hanks, N. Cherny and K. Calman), Oxford University Press, Oxford.

Shearsmith-Farthing, K. (2001) The management of altered body image: A role for occupational therapy. *British Journal of Occupational Therapy*, **64**(8), 387–92.

RECOMMENDED READING

Dougherty, L. and Lister, S. (2004) *The Royal Marsden Hospital Manual of Clinical Nursing Procedures*, 6th edn, Blackwell Science, Oxford.

Gleave, J. R. W. and MacFarlane, R. (2002) Cauda equina syndrome: What is the relationship between timing of surgery and outcome? *British Journal of Neurosurgery*, **16**(4), 325–8.

Healey, J. H. and Brown, H. K. (2000) Complications of bone metastases. *Cancer*, **88**(Suppl), 2940–51.

Thomas, S. and Mengham, H. (2002) *Eating for Health in Care Homes: A practical nutrition handbook*, Royal Institute of Public Health, London.

4 Occupational Therapy in Anxiety Management and Relaxation

JILL COOPER

WHAT IS ANXIETY?

Anxiety is a normal biological defence mechanism warning the body of potential danger and allowing it to react quickly in times of stress (Cooper, 2002). Individuals with cancer or other life-threatening illnesses may feel out of control because they have the diagnosis imposed on them, have to comply with toxic treatments that make them feel ill, and all these factors can spiral into episodes of anxiety.

Anxiety affects the body physically and symptoms may be experienced such as tensed muscles, rapid heart beat, difficulties breathing, chest pains, sweating, dizziness, nausea, dry mouth, blurred vision or frequency in micturition. Anxiety also affects the thoughts, often resulting in negative thinking. This can include thoughts such as imagining the disease is progressing, that one is having a heart attack, worrying about appearing foolish or thinking that one is going mad, and generally feeling helpless and out of control. The physical and cognitive components may combine to influence behaviour, which is affected by our thoughts and actions. Anxiety-induced behaviours can include avoiding situations or people, poor concentration, irritability, clumsiness, aggression and irregular sleep patterns and altered bowel/urinary habits.

WHAT IS STRESS?

Although it is normal for us to react to anxiety and stressful factors, such as jumping back to avoid being knocked over by a car, anxiety can become a problem when there is no obvious physical danger, but the anxiety and stress reactions are activated in the body, stopping the individual from carrying out everyday activities. Stress is an everyday occurrence and provides the stimulus to motivate us to get up, get dressed and carry out tasks. It is unavoidable and

Occupational Therapy in Oncology and Palliative Care. Edited by J. Cooper
© 2006 John Wiley & Sons Ltd

essential to our daily routines but it is how we respond that determines the impact on our lives.

Causes of stress for patients can be:

- environmental, such as noise on the ward or at home as well as the constant assault on the senses all around us;
- social, such as demands from the family and visitors, the change in dignity and privacy that people face when being treated in the healthcare system;
- physiological, such as poor health, interrupted sleep pattern, reaction to treatment as well as the illness itself;
- and thoughts, such as the worries, fears, and concerns that bombard the mind at stressful times.

THE EMERGENCY RESPONSE

When the body senses a threat, the cerebral cortex sends an alarm to the hypothalamus which stimulates the sympathetic nervous system to make a number of changes to the body. If these reactions are left unchecked and the response continues, it can have long-term negative effects (Davis *et al.*, 1999).

The brain is alerted, there is stimulation of the adrenal glands, release of corticoids into the blood stream and unpleasant symptoms that inhibit digestion, reproduction, growth and tissue repair. Consequently, it might result in vomiting or diarrhoea.

PHYSICAL SYMPTOMS OF ANXIETY AND STRESS

As part of our evolution, human beings have retained some of the reactions which their ancestors would have needed while hunting and generally surviving in prehistoric times. An example of the caveman either fleeing or fighting its prey is often used, when he would fight to kill or fight for his life, or flee for his life. Mankind still retains these physiological reactions in times of stress. It is likely that the anxious individual experiences some or all of the following symptoms:

- Headaches and dizziness are caused by the brain sending a biochemical message to the pituitary gland which releases a hormone that triggers the adrenal gland to release adrenaline. Headaches are caused by the constriction of the blood vessels in the head and neck as blood flowed to the muscles in preparation for 'fight or flight'.

- Blurred vision is the result of dilation of the pupils, which is a reaction to the hormone release.
- Palpitations and chest pain are caused by breathing becoming faster and shallower, supplying more oxygen to the muscles so that the caveman was ready for running or fighting.
- Dry mouth and difficulty swallowing are caused by body fluid such as saliva being redirected into the blood stream.
- Aching muscles, particularly the neck, head and back are the direct result of the large muscles of the body tensing themselves in readiness for action.
- Excessive sweating or blushing is caused by the body cooling itself by perspiring. Blood vessels and capillaries move close to the skin's surface to release heat.
- Rapid breathing is the result of the body attempting to supply more oxygen to the muscles.
- Tingly skin is caused by excess oxygen being supplied to the muscles as well as calcium being released from tense muscles.
- Frequent urination/diarrhoea is caused by relaxation of the bladder and sphincter muscles.

It should be emphasized that all of these physical changes are normal for an individual to experience when under a perceived threat, and that they should diminish once the individual manages to regain a feeling of safety and control.

COGNITIVE SYMPTOMS OF ANXIETY AND STRESS

The patient is likely to require help in identifying which of the anxiety-provoking situations are likely to be exacerbated as a result of negative thought patterns. Negative thought patterns may include:

- all-or-nothing thinking, when one considers oneself to be hopeless after one failed attempt at a task;
- catastrophizing, where the perception of the importance or magnitude of an event is exaggerated in the individual's opinion;
- personalizing, which involves allocating self-responsibility for unpleasant external events;
- focusing negatively, when one focuses on weaknesses, forgetting about strengths;
- jumping to conclusions, in which one predicts negatively the future without any certain facts;
- living by fixed rules when one removes the locus of control from self, thus leading to unnecessary guilt and disappointment.

BEHAVIOURAL SYMPTOMS OF ANXIETY AND STRESS

A pattern of anxious behaviour can develop with physical symptoms feeding on anxiety-provoking thoughts and vice versa until it becomes what is known as the anxiety spiral. The anxiety spiral (Figure 4.1) emphasizes what happens and how avoidance behaviour and panic attacks can occur.

Understanding this help the individuals' mind to focus on the experience that they may be undergoing in some situations, and this gives them a greater understanding and opportunity for managing the anxiety that they may feel is controlling them. Avoidance behaviour is not an effective solution to anxiety as it will become restrictive and can have a huge impact on lifestyle.

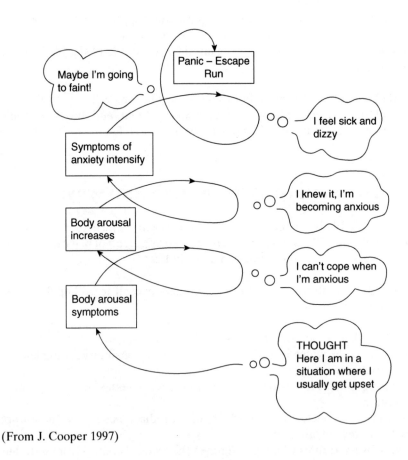

(From J. Cooper 1997)

Figure 4.1 Anxiety spiral

OCCUPATIONAL THERAPY INTERVENTION IN ANXIETY AND STRESS MANAGEMENT

THE MANAGEMENT OF THE STRESS RESPONSE

Stress management includes relaxation amongst its strategies. When the emergency response becomes a chronic learned pattern of behaviour, individuals need to learn how to counteract this response to regain control over their feelings. In order to control anxiety, the occupational therapist needs to explain to the individual what is happening, including the physiological, cognitive and behavioural reactions. Once this is understood and the person realizes that it is a normal reaction, techniques can be taught to counteract these. Stress management is not one specific treatment programme, but a general approach aimed at helping people learn new and adaptive ways of coping (Hindley and Johnston, 1999).

ASSESSMENT

A baseline of the physical, cognitive and behavioural symptoms of the individuals' anxiety needs to be identified, the assessment covering issues that make them feel anxious, the physical symptoms that arise, the thoughts involved, what action they take when this occurs and which activities create anxiety. Appendix 6 shows the occupational therapy Anxiety Management Assessment. This enables the occupational therapist to explain the anxiety reaction and why the specific individual is experiencing the difficulties.

INDIVIDUAL PERSONAL PLAN

The aim of the stress management approach is to break the spiral at an early stage using techniques such as breathing exercises and relaxation to alleviate the physical symptoms, and positive phrases to challenge the negative thoughts. The use of goal setting to break down the anxiety-provoking tasks into achievable steps is also useful in reducing anxiety symptoms and, therefore, overcoming avoidance behaviour. Each of these techniques is incorporated as part of the individual's personal plan, see Appendix 7.

CONTROLLING OVERBREATHING

Appendix 8 on a simple breathing technique gives advice for controlling overbreathing and the occupational therapist needs to explain that the breathing rate in people who feel stressed often increases. When it increases to the point that it interferes with normal bodily functioning it is called hyperventilation. This can be resolved by:

- identifying that acute hyperventilation is common during panic attacks as the body perceives a need for it in order to prepare the muscles for 'fight or flight'. When the extra O_2 that is absorbed during hyperventilation is not required by the body, it can result in frightening symptoms already discussed;
- understanding that overbreathing results in upsetting the balance of O_2/ CO_2 in the body. This makes the blood more alkaline, which then causes the unpleasant symptoms. If individuals feel more distressed due to these symptoms, they may overbreathe further, which can exacerbate the problem. Hence the spiral of overbreathing occurs.

CHALLENGING NEGATIVE THINKING

Appendix 9 on Challenging Negative Thinking shows a simple chart for challenging negative thinking, in which patients identify their thoughts when they are feeling anxious, whether or not the thoughts are reasonable and, if not, why not, and how the thoughts could be perceived in a more positive way. When this chart is filled in the occupational therapist may explain why negative thought patterns are unhelpful and can advise patients that positive alternatives will be included in their personal plan. The occupational therapist works with the individual over a period of time to challenge negative and irrational thoughts about situations and aims to replace them with positive, realistic ones. The key challenges include:

- Am I predicting the future negatively?
- What is the evidence for and against this thought?
- What would other people think in this situation?
- If things do not turn out exactly right, does it really matter?
- Is the thought helping me succeed?
- Am I making things sound worse than they are?

Guidance should be given to replace unhelpful thoughts such as 'must', 'should', 'ought' and 'what if', with 'I choose to ...' This is less demanding, more self-empowering and does not set patients up for failure with unrealistic expectations.

POSITIVE PHRASES FOR STRESSFUL ACTIVITIES

It is helpful to discuss the manner in which positive thoughts can act to relieve unwanted physical symptoms of anxiety. People can learn to 'turn off the adrenaline switch' in their body by the way they think. In doing so, individuals can learn to overcome the problems experienced as part of the anxiety spiral. By identifying 'fear conquering phrases', individuals can prepare for, confront, engage in and analyse anxiety-provoking situations. A few examples of each are listed below.

- Preparation: 'There is nothing to worry about'; 'I have succeeded with this before'; 'I will be all right.'
- Confronting: 'Take it easy step by step. Don't rush'; 'I can do this. I am doing it now'; 'It is OK to make mistakes, I will do my best'; 'I have survived this feeling before. It will go soon'; 'There is nothing to be frightened of. I am really OK.'
- Looking back: 'I did it'; 'Next time I will not have so much to worry about'; 'It is possible NOT to be scared. All I have to do is stop thinking I am scared.'

However, the best stress coping thoughts are the ones that patients write themselves. The occupational therapist works with the individuals over time to develop and list stress coping phrases that work for them. These should be included as part of the personal plan.

RELAXATION TECHNIQUES TO ASSIST WITH ANXIETY MANAGEMENT

Relaxation is a valuable aspect of anxiety management in controlling the physical symptoms and thus the mental processes and consequent behaviour. It is important to explain the link between emotional anxiety and physical tension. The body can respond to anxiety-provoking situations and thoughts with physical symptoms, e.g. muscle tension, and this, in turn, can exacerbate these anxious thoughts and the subjective experience of anxiety. The occupational therapist needs to be aware that it will take time and possibly further sessions to introduce the individuals to techniques and to identify which one(s) they find most useful, and that choosing a relaxation technique is very individualized. The occupational therapist should try to provide as broad an experience as possible and offer a wide selection. Like any exercise, relaxation is most successful if practised and if CDs are available to allow the individual to practise the techniques at home.

RELAXATION TECHNIQUES

Cooper (2002) describes the aims of relaxation as:

- to understand and recognize your level of anxiety;
- to understand the need for relaxation and recognize certain situations that may trigger tension;
- to experience a variety of relaxation techniques thus enabling you to choose the most appropriate one;
- to appreciate the importance of planning time for relaxation as part of your daily activities and lifestyle;
- to improve quality of sleep;

- to lessen pain caused by inappropriate muscle tension;
- to encourage peace of mind;
- to improve performance of physical skills;
- to increase self-esteem and confidence;
- to ease relationships with others;
- to channel and control effects of anxiety;
- to avoid unnecessary fatigue.

As with all occupational therapy intervention, thorough assessment and treatment programmes must be planned. Relaxation and stress management can be either individual sessions or in a group, but group members may have varied and diverse needs so the dynamics must be carefully considered and managed. Clear therapeutic aims and objectives are required to ensure that the patients do not develop a dependency on the occupational therapist. Relaxation techniques should be taught so that individuals can learn them and use them in their daily lives as part of a stress management approach to dealing with anxiety (Woods and Hawkins, 2002). It is vital that patients understand what is being offered in the relaxation programme, how long the programme lasts and where to continue the exercises if the individual wishes to persevere with them. Appendices 10, Relaxation Programme Assessment, and 11, Relaxation Feedback Form, illustrate the occupational therapy relaxation programme, together with Appendices 12 and 13 giving examples of relaxation scripts.

The relaxation aims are set out clearly above and cannot claim to affect the outcome of the treatment, for example, whether it helps cure cancer. It can, however, aim to help with some symptoms. A study to compare the effectiveness of Jacobson's progressive relaxation (1974), Mitchell's simple physiological relaxation and a control condition of supine lying indicated that both relaxation techniques produced significant reductions in heart rate (1987), respiratory rate and systolic and diastolic blood pressure and that neither technique was superior to the other. The control condition of supine lying produced significant reductions in heart rate and respiratory rate alone (Salt and Kerr, 1997). Autogenic relaxation techniques are discussed by Wright et al. (2002), Sahler et al. (2003), and Hidderley and Holt (2004), the results of which indicate improved quality of life with oncology and palliative care patients.

Sloman (2002) reported in a study of 56 patients treated with imagery and progressive muscular relaxation that there was no actual significant improvement for anxiety but significant positive changes occurred for depression and quality of life. Schultz (2001) described a group of women with primary breast carcinoma experiencing psychosocial problems and concluded that progressive muscular relaxation reduced psychological distress for them. Molassiotis (2000) reported on a pilot study in which this training was an effective adjuvant method in decreasing nausea and vomiting in chemotherapy patients.

SUMMARY

Occupational therapy intervention assesses the presenting problems and explores the meaning of the symptoms to the individual and the impact on that individual and the family. The occupational therapist needs to ask, 'What does this problem stop people from doing?'

By carrying out the treatment programme, the occupational therapist enables and facilitates the individual in taking back some control over their physical and psychological feelings, and helps them and their carers to cope with the anxiety. The goals need to be led by the individual. The individuals' are acknowledged and clear therapeutic aims are set to work towards improved quality of life and reduced anxiety.

ACTION POINTS

1. A person is referred to occupational therapy for relaxation. Consider the approach taken by the occupational therapist in contacting this individual and how the treatment programme would be explained to them.
2. How would the occupational therapist address the problem of the patient who wishes to continue seeing the occupational therapist weekly for relaxation and does not want to be discharged after the relaxation programme has been completed?
3. Explore the different techniques used in anxiety management and relaxation and how these can be applied to different individuals.

REFERENCES

Cooper, J. (1997) *Occupational Therapy in Oncology and Palliative Care*, Whurr, London.

Cooper, J. (2002) Oncology. *Occupational Therapy and Physical Dysfunction* (eds A. Turner, M. Foster and S. E. Johnson), Churchill Livingstone, Edinburgh.

Davis, M., Robbins Eschelman, E. and McKay, M. (1999) *The Relaxation and Stress Reduction Workbook*, New Harbinger Publications Inc, Oakland, CA.

Hidderley, M. and Holt, M. (2004) A pilot randomized trial assessing the effects of autogenic training in early stage cancer patients in relation to psychological status and immune system responses. *European Journal of Oncology Nursing*, 8(1), 61–5.

Hindley, M. and Johnston, S. (1999) Stress management for breast cancer patients: Service development. *International Journal of Palliative Nursing*, 5(3), 135–41.

Jacobson, E. (1974) *Progressive Relaxation*, University of Chicago Press, Chicago.

Mitchell, L. (1987) *Simple Relaxation: the Mitchell method of physiological relaxation for easing tension*. Murray, London.

Molassiotis, A. (2000) A pilot study of the use of progressive muscular relaxation training in the management of post-chemotherapy nausea and vomiting. *European Journal of Cancer Care*, 9(4), 230–4.

Sahler, O. J. Z., Hunterm, B. C. and Liesveld, J. L. (2003) The effect of using music therapy with relaxation imagery in the management of patients undergoing bone marrow transplantation: A pilot feasibility study. *Alternative Therapies in Health and Medicine*, **9**(6), 70–4.

Salt, V. L. and Kerr, K. M. (1997) Mitchell's simple physiological relaxation and Jacobson's progressive relaxation techniques: A comparison. *Physiotherapy*, **83**(4), 200–7.

Schultz, K. (2001) A psychosocial group intervention reduced psychological distress and enhanced coping in primary breast cancer. *Evidence-Based Mental Health*, **4**(1), 15.

Sloman, R. (2002) Relaxation and imagery for anxiety and depression control in community patients with advanced cancer. *Cancer Nursing*, **25**(6), 432–5.

Woods, S. and Hawkins, C. (2002) HIV/AIDS, in *Occupational Therapy and Physical Dysfunction* (eds A. Turner, M. Foster and S. E. Johnson), Churchill Livingstone, Edinburgh.

Wright, S., Courtney, U. and Crowther, D. (2002) A quantitative and qualitative pilot study of the perceived benefits of autogenic training for a group of people with cancer. *European Journal of Cancer Care*, **11**(2), 122–30.

SUGGESTED READING

Ewer-Smith, C. and Patterson, S. (2002) The use of an occupational therapy programme within a palliative care setting. *European Journal of Palliative Care*, **9**(1), 30–3.

Keable, D. (1997) *The Management of Anxiety – Client Packs*, Churchill Livingstone, Edinburgh.

Payne, R. A. (1995) *Relaxation Techniques: A practical handbook for the health care professional*. Churchill Livingstone, Edinburgh.

Powell, T. (2001) *The Mental Health Handbook*, Speechmark Publishing Ltd, Bicester.

5 Occupational Therapy in the Management of Breathlessness

JILL COOPER

WHAT IS BREATHLESSNESS?

Breathlessness, or dyspnoea, is the term generally applied to unpleasant or uncomfortable respiratory sensations experienced by individuals (Chan *et al.*, 2004). Breathing is an automatic activity that takes place effortlessly for many people throughout their lives, expressing physiological, psychological and spiritual signals depending on the level of activity and mood. For individuals with advanced disease affecting the lungs, breathing can become distressed and laborious. As with other symptoms experienced by patients in advanced stages of disease, difficulty with breathing is a subjective and personal experience and means different things to different people. It can be exacerbated by fatigue and anxiety, limit function and restrict normal activity. It can be described as ranging from tightness in the chest, needing to gasp or pant to extreme fear or 'suffocation' or 'drowning' (Cooper, 2002). Factors relating to prevalence of breathlessness are:

- site of the primary disease, mainly lung, breast and colorectal;
- metastases to lung or pleura;
- lung irradiation;
- past history of cardiac or pulmonary diseases;
- low performance status;
- smoking;
- exposure to asbestos, coal, cotton and grain dust.

Intensity of this symptom depends on:

- lung involvement, whether it is primary or secondary;
- metastases to mediastinum, hila or ribs;

- anxiety;
- fatigue or tiredness;
- vital capacity;
- maximum inspiratory pressure.

(Chan *et al.*, 2004)

ASSESSMENT

Whether the underlying causes of breathlessness are due to advanced heart disease, chronic respiratory disease or advanced cancer, the complex presentation of breathlessness requires thorough assessment to ensure appropriate medical treatment is initiated. The symptom may be caused by a tumour, by treatment for the malignancy, be linked to general failing health or be the result of other pre-existing disease (Hately *et al.*, 2001). Specific causes of breathlessness can include:

- chronic obstructive pulmonary disease (COPD), experienced by 37–50% of cancer patients, individuals with chronic bronchitis and emphysema, asthma, bronchiectasis, and cystic fibrosis;
- restrictive disease including interstitial lung diseases such as fibrosing alveolitis, sarcoidosis, asbestosis and neuromuscular/skeletal disorders resulting in ankylosing spondylitis (Oliver and Sewell, 2002);
- superior vena cava syndrome, in which the primary cancer may be lung, lymphoma, breast or solid tumours;
- obstruction of bronchus, caused by collapse of the pulmonary parenchyma lower to the occlusion with possible infection;
- carcinomatous lymphangitis, severe and continuous dyspnoea with minimal physical and radiological findings;
- pleural effusion, with dyspnoea, unproductive cough, chest pain, caused by lung, breast, ovarian, gastric cancers, lymphoma or leukaemia;
- pericardial effusion when there is decreased cardiac output and severe shortness of breath, with or without cardiac tamponade (Ripamonti, 1999).

OCCUPATIONAL THERAPY ROLE IN THE MANAGEMENT OF BREATHLESSNESS

The occupational therapist works as part of the multiprofessional team to help the patient cope with the symptoms (Syrett and Taylor, 2003). The highest proportion of breathless patients have a diagnosis of primary lung/bronchus, colorectal and breast cancers (Vainio and Auvinen, 1996). There is no recipe for the occupational therapy approach in the management of breathlessness as patients will have their unique difficulties and fears, and there is no quick-fix solution to the problems. As with other symptom management, the occupational therapist needs to take a problem-solving approach, which is likely to require several sessions over a period of time to establish rapport and confidence.

The occupational therapy approach aims to:

- explore meaning of the symptom to the patients and their carers and families;
- enable activity so that they can achieve optimum independence and control despite this debilitating symptom;
- help patients manage any anxiety and panic attacks, including teaching relaxation techniques as part of the management programme.

EXPLORING MEANING

Triggers

The occupational therapist works with the patient to identify 'triggers' that initiate episodes of breathlessness and that exacerbate these episodes. This is particularly pertinent to occupational therapy when undertaking activity makes breathlessness worse.

Fears

The patients' fears need to be explored so that the occupational therapist can help them recognize what the breathlessness signifies to them. This can then be addressed in anxiety and panic management.

Patterns

Once the triggers and fears are established, patterns of breathlessness can then be looked at to establish when the symptom occurs, when it worsens and what is affecting it.

Role changes

It is important within the occupational therapy assessment to establish how breathlessness is impacting on individuals and those around them, how it is affecting their involvement in family life, work and social life.

Effect on family and carers

By involving the carers in the assessment and treatment sessions, they can all work together to learn coping strategies for the management of breathlessness.

ENABLING ACTIVITY

Analysis of activities

By analysing activities that exacerbate the symptom of breathlessness, the occupational therapist has the unique skill of being able to break down and analyse the movements and underlying psychological fears. These can then be addressed with possible solutions, including changing techniques of actually carrying out the activities, adapting the activity itself and providing equipment to facilitate physical effort.

Strategies

The development of coping strategies should appear to be a seamless part of the occupational therapy approach alongside the assessment. Once the elements of the patient's lifestyle and the problems they are encountering with the breathlessness are established, the strategies known as the 5 'P's as seen in Appendix 15 can be introduced. These can be reinforced by all healthcare professionals in the multiprofessional team as they cover all aspects of everyday life in the 'prioritizing, planning, pacing, positioning and permission'.

Assessing the home environment

The occupational therapist can help advise on adapting and rearranging the individual's home environment to minimize the effects of breathlessness. This may involve access to the property, whether the front or back doorstep needs altering to make it physically easier to manage or whether a rail is required that would facilitate getting in and out of the property.

All transfers and activities can be assessed, but this should take place over several visits to avoid assessment becoming too tiring for the patient. Heights of furniture, bathing, shower, toilet aids/commode, stair rails and other equipment to aid daily living can be introduced, *but at all times the occupational therapist must remember not to overload the individual with too much clutter.*

Aids and adaptations

The occupational therapy interventions should be introduced gradually as and when the patient feels ready to accept them. There are dozens of items in catalogues that can help alleviate physical exertion and a range of different techniques to manage activities less energetically. The occupational therapist must assess when it is appropriate to introduce any of these interventions, always bearing in mind the psychological and emotional impact as well as the physical benefits.

MANAGING ANXIETY AND PANIC ATTACKS

Education

Learning breathing techniques and how to pace activity, balancing exertion with rest, is as vital as the need for psychological support (Syrett and Taylor, 2003). Chapter 4 explains the principles of anxiety management and relaxation. The individual is likely to be terrified by the experience of breathlessness, and this exacerbates the symptom, thus becoming a vicious circle or spiral of anxiety as seen in Figure 4.1 (see p. 44). Oliver and Sewell (2002) describe a downward spiral of disability, with the physical impairment of breathlessness spiralling downwards from fear of breathlessness, to decreased activity, decreased tolerance to activity and associated muscle atrophy, to an increased level of fatigue. This then leads down to deconditioning, loss of function, social isolation and loss of role, status and function, which results in the individual becoming disabled and debilitated by the breathlessness.

All of the multiprofessional team must, therefore, have a consistent approach to encourage the patients to incorporate anxiety management into their daily routine whenever possible, to be able to cope with the panic and break the spirals of anxiety and disability. Griffiths *et al.* (2000) advised that pulmonary or cardiac rehabilitation programmes that reinforce the message that being breathless is a normal consequence of exertion have found that people's negative perceptions of breathlessness can diminish.

Strategies to regain control

Appendix 16 is a simple personal plan for patients to identify which position they find most helpful to alleviate the breathlessness, the methods they have found most useful to relax their shoulders and upper chest, and the techniques they find assist in calming their breathing. All of these can be completed over a period of time with input from the occupational therapist, physiotherapist and nursing staff whether at home or in hospital, and these can be changed as the patient develops expertise in coping. The techniques to regain control and relaxation techniques may also change as the patient's condition changes. Appendix 17 shows simple advice to supplement occupational therapy and other team members' treatment sessions.

Goal setting

The occupational therapist can use clear measurable and achievable goals with patients to help them identify what they would like to manage. Goal setting also shows patients how they have coped using the strategies and is a tool to build on positive perceptions. Even if the breathlessness deteriorates with disease progression, this situation can be addressed honestly, enabling the patient to cope with the change in circumstances by using different strategies.

PROBLEM-SOLVING APPROACH OF
OCCUPATIONAL THERAPY

As well as the practical coping strategies as identified in Appendices 15–17, Oliver and Sewell (2002) discuss a more detailed problem-solving approach by occupational therapy in the management of breathlessness, as follows:

SENSATION OF BREATHLESSNESS

As discussed above, the physical reaction to the feeling of being out of control can be addressed by educating the patient that this is a normal sensation given the disease process. The social isolation resulting from the symptom requires a more detailed discussion with the individual regarding their belief system, how it is impacting on their lives and how that makes them feel. Exploration of the individual's understanding of the mechanisms of breathing can help in addressing reduced tolerance to activity and the anxiety and depression that may occur. This approach can lead to the introduction of an activity programme which can increase duration of activity balancing demand (physical and mental tolerance to activity) and effect (level of fatigue, breathlessness and anxiety).

EXPECTATION OF SELF REALIZING THE GULF BETWEEN HOPES, ASPIRATIONS AND REALITY OF LOSS

The patient may be experiencing reduced motivation, grief and low self-esteem, which the occupational therapist can acknowledge and address by using graded therapeutic activities to encourage motivation and enjoyment. Activities of daily living can be adapted to focus intervention on what can be achieved, and relaxation techniques used to reduce tension and promote well-being.

EXPECTATION OF OTHERS

The patient may feel guilty at being unable to have a 'normal' relationship, be resentful of those with good health, have reduced understanding of their disease and there may be conflict between the individual and carers. The occupational therapist as part of the multiprofessional team needs to encourage good communication of their fears to 'normalize' the situation and neutralize the stigma of illness. The family and carers require education about the mechanism of breathing and consequences of being breathless. By acknowledging and validating any conflict, it may reduce the impact on the individual and those around them. Again, relaxation for all those involved may be of benefit.

ISOLATION OF TRIGGER FACTORS

It is important to identify triggers, as avoidance of them may result in ritualistic behaviour, social isolation and reduced capacity for fulfilling occupations. In order to prevent maladaptive behaviour, positive behaviour patterns need to be encouraged, for example, 'the individual believes that if he does not get dressed then he will not become breathless' could be replaced with techniques of breaking down the activity to facilitate getting dressed without becoming breathless. Graded programmes can be introduced with a variety of activities to increase well-being and ability to cope with varying levels of breathlessness and fatigue. Good posture can be reinforced to eliminate unnecessary breathlessness and maintenance of environmental factors such as good ventilation and temperature control may help.

QUESTIONING OF OWN MORTALITY

The patient is likely to lack assurance that the body is working efficiently which requires an honest and supportive approach by the whole team to enable the grief process and adaption to the diagnosis. It is perfectly reasonable for the individual and carers to feel that the disease cannot be cured, that they are losing control and are helpless, the situation is hopeless because of the lack of choice and there are no options so making them feel useless. The occupational therapist along with the multiprofessional team must, again, use an honest and supportive approach to look at enabling the individual to seek meaning in life through participation in purposeful occupation and activities if they wish to. Redefinition of roles can still enable the individual to lead a fulfilling life and help can be given to set goals and achieve these however small they may be.

(Oliver and Sewell, 2002.
Reproduced by kind permission of Elsevier Ltd.)

A study was carried out to evaluate the effectiveness of occupational therapy as an adjunctive measuring during pulmonary rehabilitation. In the programme consisting of 18 three-hour daily sessions, occupational therapy (domestic activities) was added and concluded that the addition of occupational therapy to the comprehensive programme was able to specifically improve the outcome of severely disabled patients with chronic obstructive pulmonary disease (Lorenzi *et al.*, 2004). Ripamonti (1999) studied the management of breathlessness in patients with advanced cancer and concluded that 'other components of the symptom expression are better managed by supportive counselling, occupational therapy and physiotherapy.' Tucakovic *et al.* (2001) studied gynaecological malignancies affecting the respiratory system both directly and indirectly and stated that patients needed non-pharmacological therapies including energy conservation, home redesign, relief strategies, relaxation and attention to spiritual suffering.

Breathlessness can be an exhausting and potentially terrifying symptom for palliative care patients and a collaborative approach enables professionals and patients to share expertise and work towards their common goal (Syrett and Taylor, 2003). The patients and carers of those with breathlessness need support, education and explanations, training in coping strategies and prompt intervention to optimize functional activities.

SUMMARY

Corner *et al.* (1996) state that 'The emotional experience of breathlessness cannot be separated from the sensory experience and biological mechanism. Non-pharmalogical strategies improve considerably the patient's ability to self-care and reduce the levels of perceived breathlessness and distress.' Bredin *et al.*'s research (1999) concluded that 'Interventions based on a range of strategies combining psychosocial support, breathing control, activity pacing and relaxation techniques can help patients to experience improvements in breathlessness, performance status and reduce physical and emotional distress.'

Each patient will be experiencing different problems, and whereas the occupational therapist will have a breadth of knowledge of techniques and equipment which worked for other patients, it must be reiterated that there is no recipe for success with this symptom. Not all physical problems caused by breathlessness, such as bath transfers, can be solved by providing equipment to aid transfers, as this might not be the fundamental problem as perceived by the individual. The occupational therapist must analyse and assess each individual and establish appropriate solutions with them. All of this needs to be introduced sensitively to individuals as any equipment may be another visual reminder of their illness and may need to be promoted as a means of retaining independence rather than a mark of dependence.

ACTION POINTS

1. Consider the functional implications of breathlessness for a younger individual compared to those for an older person and the impact of their lifestyles, roles and the family whom they may have around them.

2. How would you liaise with other members of the multiprofessional team in assessing and treating the individual with breathlessness in order to avoid repetition of questions and the burden of assessment on the patient?
3. If the patient has a very poor prognosis and is requesting assessment for a major adaptation, for example, stair lift at home, how would you address this request given a possible lack of resources in your social services? What might you advise as an alternative to help the person manage more comfortably and independently at home?

REFERENCES

Bredin, M., Corner, J., Krishnasamy, M., Plant, H., Bailey, C. and A'Hern, R. (1999) Multicentre randomised controlled trial of nursing intervention for breathlessness in patients with lung cancer. *British Medical Journal*, **318**(7188), 888–9.

Chan, K-S., Sham, M. M. K., Tse, D. M. W. and Thorsen, A. B. (2004) Palliative medicine in malignant respiratory diseases. *Oxford Textbook of Palliative Medicine*, 3rd edn (eds D. Doyle, G. Hanks, N. Cherny and K. Calman), Oxford University Press, Oxford.

Cooper, J. (2002) Oncology. *Occupational Therapy and Physical Dysfunction*, 5th edn (eds A. Turner, M. Foster and S. E. Johnson), Churchill Livingstone, Edinburgh.

Corner, J., Plant, H., A'Hern, R. and Bailey, C. (1996) Non-pharmacological intervention for breathlessness in lung cancer. *Palliative Medicine*, **10**(4), 299–305.

Griffiths, T. L., Burr, M. L. and Campbell, I. A. (2000) Results at 1 year of outpatient multidisciplinary pulmonary rehabilitation: A randomised trial. *Lancet*, **355**(9201), 362–8.

Hately, J., Scott, A., Laurence, V., Baker, R. and Thomas, P. (2001) A palliative-care approach for breathlessness in cancer: A clinical evaluation. *Lewis-Manning House Cancer Trust*, Help the Hospices, London.

Lorenzi, C. M., Cilione, C., Rizzardi, R., Furino, V., Bellantone, T., Lugli, D. and Clini, E. (2004) Occupational therapy and pulmonary rehabilitation of disabled COPD patients. *Respiration*, **71**(3), 246–51.

Oliver, K. and Sewell, L. (2002) Cardiac and respiratory disease. *Occupational Therapy and Physical Dysfunction*, 5th edn (eds A. Turner, M. Foster and S. E. Johnson), Churchill Livingstone, Edinburgh.

Ripamonte, C. (1999) Management of dyspnea in advanced cancer patients. *Support Care Cancer*, **7**(4), 233–43.

Syrett, E. and Taylor, J. (2003) Non-pharmacological management of breathlessness: A collaborative nurse-physiotherapist approach. *International Journal of Palliative Nursing*, **9**(4), 150–6.

Tucakovic, M., Bascom, R. and Bascom, P. B. (2001) Pulmonary medicine and palliative care. *Best Practice and Research. Clinical Obstetrics and Gynaecology*, **15**(2), 291–304.

Vainio, A. and Auvinen, A. (1996) Prevalence of symptoms among patients with advanced cancer: An international collaborative study. *Journal of Pain and Symptom Management*, **12**(1), 3–10.

RECOMMENDED READING

www.roycastle.org
www.bbc.co.uk/health
www.cancerbacup.org.uk
www.cancerguide.org
www.lungcancer.org

6 Occupational Therapy and Cancer-Related Fatigue

DANIEL LOWRIE

Fatigue is recognized as being the most frequently experienced and distressing symptom of cancer and its treatment, affecting between 70% and 100% of people with cancer (Ahlberg *et al.*, 2003). For many patients the problems associated with cancer-related fatigue can continue months or even years after their treatment is finished. Despite this the mechanisms that cause cancer-related fatigue remain poorly understood (Wagner and Cella, 2004) and the evidence base regarding many approaches to fatigue management utilized by healthcare professionals is not strong (Ahlberg *et al.*, 2003).

Ream and Richardson (1996) describe the concept of fatigue as 'a subjective, unpleasant symptom which incorporates total body feelings ranging from tiredness to exhaustion creating an unrelenting overall condition which interferes with individual's ability to function to their normal capacity.' Fatigue in cancer is defined by the National Comprehensive Cancer Network (Mock *et al.*, 2004) as 'a persistent, subjective sense of tiredness related to cancer or cancer treatment that interferes with usual functioning.'

Based on these descriptions of cancer-related fatigue, and taking into account their emphasis on the impact of fatigue on function, it is clear that occupational therapists have a valuable role to play in the management of fatigue in cancer. The client-centred and holistic approach to rehabilitation and problem-solving skills of occupational therapists enables them to work collaboratively with patients to assess fatigue and develop strategies for its management specific to individual patients' needs.

This chapter will discuss the causes and effects of cancer-related fatigue and approaches to its assessment and management. It will focus on the unique role of the occupational therapist in ensuring best outcomes for patients experiencing difficulty with this symptom.

CAUSES OF FATIGUE IN CANCER

As stated earlier the exact physiological mechanisms that cause cancer-related fatigue are not known. It is hypothesized that there is an interrelationship

Occupational Therapy in Oncology and Palliative Care. Edited by J. Cooper
© 2006 John Wiley & Sons Ltd

between multiple physiological and psychosocial causes which compound each other and result in the complex presentation of fatigue in people with cancer (Wagner and Cella, 2004).

Ahlberg *et al.* (2003) reviewed the current literature concerning the causes of cancer-related fatigue. They suggest that the physiological causes of cancer-related fatigue may include:

- anaemia;
- effects of cancer treatments (e.g. radiotherapy, chemotherapy, hormonal therapy);
- cachexia (reduced hunger as a result of increased cytokine production, and loss of nutrients due to anorexia, nausea, vomiting or hypermetabolism);
- tumour burden (size, site and stage of tumour, extent of metastatic disease);
- increased production of cytokines (proteins involved in the generation of an immune response).

It is unclear whether the psychosocial factors that have been associated with cancer-related fatigue are causes, effects or both, of the symptom. However, the psychosocial factors that have been found to have a positive correlation with fatigue in cancer are summarized by Ahlberg *et al.* (2003) as including:

- anxiety and depression;
- sleeping difficulties;
- full-time employment status;
- reductions in physical functioning.

SYMPTOM CLUSTERS

Dodd, Miaskowski and Paul (2001) investigated the impact of groups of three or more related symptoms (symptom clusters) on the morbidity of people with cancer. They found that the combination of multiple concurrent symptoms (e.g. fatigue, pain and sleep loss) negatively impacted upon the functional status of people with cancer. Given *et al.* (2001) found that patients experiencing fatigue and pain, rather than fatigue or pain alone tend to experience much higher numbers of other co-occurring symptoms. This finding is reinforced by studies by Okuyama *et al.* (2001) and Cooley *et al.* (2003) that reported that on average people with lung cancer presented with more than four highly distressing symptoms the most common of which was fatigue. Such studies highlight the importance of occupational therapists adopting a systems approach to symptom management as it indicates that working to address one symptom (e.g. fatigue) at the exclusion of other concurrent symptoms is unlikely to result in best outcomes. They also indicate the importance of fatigue (and pain) management as a means of reducing the occurrence and severity of other symptoms of cancer.

PATTERNS OF FATIGUE IN CANCER

In order to ensure the timely screening and assessment of and preparation for the potential onset of cancer-related fatigue, it is beneficial to have an understanding of the patterns of fatigue that tend to occur depending on factors such as tumour type and stage or treatment regime. It should be remembered, however, that due to the large numbers of factors that contribute to cancer-related fatigue, knowledge of fatigue patterns is far from comprehensive, and what is known is only reflective of trends with regard to the onset, duration and severity of cancer-related fatigue and may not be representative of specific individual symptom experience. Knowledge of fatigue patterns should be used cautiously, therefore, to prompt further discussion about and analysis of the symptom with individual patients, rather than to formulate a concrete pathway for pre-determined interventions (Richardson, Ream and Wilson-Barnett, 1998).

Servaes, Verhagen and Bleijenberg (2002) report that the evidence linking cancer diagnosis and the level of fatigue is presently divided. The majority of studies report no clear relationship between primary cancer diagnosis and fatigue. Similarly, it has been suggested that stage of cancer does not correlate with people's incidence of fatigue (de Jong *et al.*, 2002; Servaes, Verhagen and Bleijenberg, 2002). Some studies note people with more advanced or metastatic disease reporting higher levels of distress caused by severe cancer-related fatigue (Stone *et al.*, 2000b; Krishnasamy, 2004). Clearly more research is required with regard to these variables before conclusions can be drawn concerning their impact upon patterns of fatigue in people with cancer.

In her review of the current literature concerning patterns of fatigue following chemotherapy Richardson (2004) identified that patterns of fatigue may differ somewhat depending on the chemotherapy regime, method and frequency of administration or due to disease-related factors. Generally however, fatigue resulting from chemotherapy has most often been observed to occur in a cyclical pattern with a peak within a few days post-treatment and then a gradual reduction up until the next treatment (Richardson, 2004). However, one study by Richardson *et al.* (1998) found an interim rise in fatigue levels around the nadir period (between treatments), which then declined again before the next cycle of treatment. Occasional occurrences of slight rises in fatigue levels prior to the commencement of chemotherapy treatments have also been reported, which it has been hypothesized may be a result of the emotional distress associated with treatment (Jacobsen *et al.*,

1999) or, in the case of subsequent chemotherapy cycles, may have an antici-patory element to it (Richardson *et al.*, 1998). Although it has been suggested in the past that fatigue from chemotherapy may be cumulative as treatment cycles progress, two studies of patients receiving chemotherapy for breast cancer (Berger, 1998; Jacobsen *et al.*, 1999) found that this did not occur. More recently, in their analysis of fatigue patterns in patients receiving chemo-therapy for breast, lung, ovarian, colorectal cancer, osteosarcoma, leukaemia or lymphoma, Kearney *et al.* (2004) reported that although the incidence of cancer-related fatigue usually remains stable across cycles of treatment, the severity of, and distress caused by, fatigue often increases as treatment progresses.

More research is required regarding the incidence of fatigue depending upon method, site and aims of radiotherapy as well as number of fractions and cumulative radiotherapy dose (Richardson, 2004). Based on existing studies Richardson (2004) states that radiotherapy-induced fatigue tends to begin on the first day of treatment and then increase cumulatively until reach-ing a plateau between the second and fourth week. Some researchers describe a reduction in the second week of treatment, which they argue may be a result of the body's natural adaptation to the effects of radiotherapy (Jereczek-Fossa, Marsiglia and Orecchia, 2002). Fatigue typically diminishes gradually once treatment is completed and generally resolves after the first three months (Richardson, 2004) although this is not always the case with patients some-times reporting the existence of fatigue long after radiotherapy has ceased (Schwartz *et al.*, 2000b).

There is currently little research investigating patterns of fatigue that result from other treatment regimes (e.g. surgical, hormonal or biological treat-ments) and as a result the precise relationship between these treatment modalities and fatigue is not clearly understood (Servaes *et al.*, 2002). Most studies that have been conducted have found fatigue to be a major problem for patients receiving these treatments. Cooley *et al.* (2003) investigated 45 adults treated surgically for lung cancer and found approximately 56% of these people experienced fatigue in the period immediately following their surgery with a gradual decline to approximately 32% after three months. In another study, significant problems with fatigue and concentration were found at two weeks and three months in women following surgery for breast cancer compared to a control group who did not have breast cancer (Cimprich and Ronis, 2001). Galloway and Graydon (1996) found fatigue to be the most distressing symptom experienced by patients following surgery for colon cancer. All symptom distress scores in this patient group were in the low range.

Stone *et al.* (2000a) investigated patients with prostate cancer following three months' treatment with first-line hormone therapy and found a similar incidence of fatigue to that of patients with the same diagnosis who underwent radical radiotherapy (approximately 66%). Fatigue in this study increased for six weeks following the commencement of treatment before then stabilizing. Fatigue was also recorded in a study of women with breast cancer who received hormonal therapy. However, patterns of fatigue were not described (Woo *et al.*, 1998).

Fatigue associated with biological therapies (such as interferon α or interleukin-2) is generally reported to be more severe than fatigue resulting from any of the other mainstream cancer treatments. It is reported to be persistent, pervasive and cumulative in nature and can on occasions be so severe as to lead patients to terminate their treatment (Porock and Juenger, 2004). In a study of 280 patients with melanoma receiving interferon, Donnelly (1998) found fatigue affected 96% of the patient group. Problems with fatigue have also been reported in patients receiving biological therapies as treatment for metastatic renal (Figlin *et al.*, 1992) and metastatic breast cancer (Madhusudan *et al.*, 2004).

Although it is evident that each of the previously mentioned treatment approaches can result in cancer-related fatigue, the combination of treatment modalities has been found to further increase fatigue severity (Woo *et al.*, 1998; Fu *et al.*, 2002; Jereczek-Fossa *et al.*, 2002). Occupational therapists should consider the potential for this when working with patients undergoing multiple treatment regimes.

EFFECTS OF CANCER-RELATED FATIGUE

There is considerable evidence that cancer-related fatigue has a major effect on people's lives. In a study of 397 patients with cancer Curt *et al.* (2000) found 301 (76%) had experienced fatigue for at least a few days during their last treatment cycle. Of these, 91% of respondents reported that their fatigue prevented them from leading a normal life. Eighty-eight percent had been forced to make alterations to their normal daily routines and 75% had needed to make changes to their employment status. Similar results have been found by Volgelzang *et al.* (1997) and Stone *et al.* (2000c) who also identified the effects of cancer-related fatigue on a number of issues including their ability to take care of their families, to enjoy life, to engage in sexual activity, to maintain meaningful relationships with family and friends, and to retain their hope of fighting their cancer.

It is clear from this that cancer-related fatigue can have diverse and profound physical, emotional, cognitive and social effects on people with cancer that impact on their functional ability and lifestyle as a whole. Occupational therapists therefore need to be holistic, dynamic and creative in their approach to assessing and addressing fatigue if the problems stemming from it are to be managed.

ASSESSING FATIGUE IN CANCER

In order for cancer-related fatigue to be well managed, thorough screening and assessment are essential (Ruckdeschel, 2005). Unfortunately, there is considerable evidence to suggest that the symptom of fatigue is frequently overlooked or under-assessed by healthcare professionals (Vogelzang *et al.*, 1997; Stone, Hardy *et al.*, 2000a). Stone, Richards *et al.* (2000b) found that despite the high prevalence and debilitating nature of fatigue in people with cancer, very few patients (approx. 14%) report that healthcare professionals offer support, treatment or advice for its management. This is despite the fact that simply being given the opportunity to talk about their fatigue with health-care professionals is recognized by many patients as being a very important strategy for its management (Krishnasamy, 1997).

It is essential, therefore, that occupational therapists incorporate discussion regarding the effects of fatigue upon their patients' lifestyles as part of their initial assessment process. This should include questions to ascertain the presence of fatigue, explore its patterns and severity and investigate its impact on activities of daily living and any strategies currently being used by the patient to try to combat these problems. Clinical assessments of fatigue should also include open dialogue and allow opportunity for patients to describe their own lived experience of fatigue and the impact it has upon them (Krishnasamy, 1997). When enquiring about the existence of fatigue, consi-deration should be given to the fact that many patients may be uncomfortable using the word fatigue and may instead prefer to use different language to describe their experiences and the meaning that they associate with the symptom (Krishnasamy, 1997; Richardson and Ream, 1998).

Fatigue diaries have been utilized by Richardson (1994), Richardson and Ream (1998) and Borthwick *et al.* (2003) as a means of objectively monitoring changes in the severity of, distress caused by and influence of fatigue on patients' lives over time. These diaries were found to be helpful in gathering information about the fatigue triggers and patterns of fatigue as well as the effectiveness of interventions used by patients. A similar approach was adopted more recently as part of the Workflow Information Systems for European Nursing Care (WISECARE+) project (Kearney *et al.*, 2004). The project involved the use of internet linked, electronic diaries used by patients undergoing chemotherapy to objectively record their fatigue, nausea and vomiting and oral problems over time. This electronically collected data was then used by staff as a quantifiable record of the person's symptom experi-ences to guide the formulation of a management plan.

Due to the ongoing and multidimensional nature of cancer-related fatigue, formal assessment should include measurement of both objective and subject-ive expressions of fatigue (Richardson, 1998). Numerous fatigue assessment tools exist, which in addition to measuring the severity of fatigue, also incorp-orate items related to its physical, behavioural, affective, cognitive, sensory and temporal dimensions (Piper, 2004). Numerous, standardized, psycho-metrically tested assessment and screening tools for cancer-related fatigue exist. Useful comparisons of the properties of different measures have been conducted by Piper (2004) and Horng-Shiuann and McSweeny (2004). When choosing an assessment tool consideration should be given to the cultural background and cognitive status of patients being assessed, as these factors may have an impact on their responses. Consideration should also be given to the potential for administrative burden that can result if lengthy assessment forms are used, as by their very nature, such processes can potentially induce or increase fatigue in some patients (Richardson, 1998).

Although the use of standardized, objective tools play an important role in the assessment of fatigue, it is very important that the benefits of task-specific functional assessments are not overlooked (Winningham, 2001). Occupational therapists are highly skilled in activity analysis and therefore can identify components of tasks compromised by problems (such as fatigue) as required to enable the development of potential solutions. Fatigue may affect activities related to people's self-care, leisure, productivity or rest, all of which should be the domain of concern of occupational therapists working in cancer care.

OCCUPATIONAL THERAPY AND THE MANAGEMENT OF CANCER-RELATED FATIGUE

To date there is little published literature providing specific, direct evidence of the role of occupational therapy in the management of fatigue in cancer. However, the key underlying principles of fatigue management that are con-sidered to constitute best practice and many of the approaches that have been found to assist in the management of the symptom sit comfortably within the theoretical framework of occupational therapy. Regardless, it remains import-ant that occupational therapists engage in and publish research demonstrating the efficacy of their interventions in the management of fatigue in cancer so that the unique role of the profession in this area can be both better under-stood and proven.

Any strategies for fatigue management recommended by occupational therapists must take into account the physical, psychological, cognitive and social dimensions of fatigue. Attempts to manage the physical components of fatigue that fail to acknowledge the psychological, cognitive or social compo-nents are unlikely to be successful. Further to this, patients' experiences of fatigue are likely to be unique and may change at different stages of the cancer journey (Richardson and Ream, 1996). As a result there is no one simple set of strategies that can be adopted to promote fatigue management and clini-cians need to work collaboratively with their patients to identify a tailored package of management strategies that are most appropriate for the patient at any given time (Barsevick *et al.*, 2002; Krishnasamy, 2004). These strategies may be aimed at reducing extent and severity of fatigue, minimizing the impact of fatigue on patients' daily lives and/or preventing and alleviating distress caused by fatigue (Ream and Stone, 2004). Information, advice and support with fatigue management may take place in sessions between the patients, their carers and the occupational therapist, as part of a multi-faceted group support programme or a combination of all.

EDUCATION

The provision of clear and timely education forms a crucial component of any programme of fatigue management. It is important that patients are informed about the likely onset of fatigue so that they can be prepared for and anticipate the patterns of fatigue that may occur as a result of the specific treatment regime that they receive (Escalante, 2003). Patients who are advised of the potential impact that fatigue may have upon them prior to its onset tend to report a less negative overall experience of their fatigue (Ream *et al.*, 2003).

When discussing cancer-related fatigue the occupational therapist should be aware that patients will have their own, pre-existing conceptual understanding of fatigue that may be markedly different from the reality of chronic cancer-related fatigue (Reuille, 2002). Patients may therefore need time to discuss issues concerning the physical, sensory, cognitive and temporal characteristics of cancer-related fatigue and the potential impact that these may have on their personal, social, vocational and recreational activities of daily living. By doing this occupational therapists can assist patients to develop strategies to overcome potential problems prior to their occurrence.

Ream *et al.* (2002) report the inclusion of an education programme for patients incorporating information about their likely experience of fatigue as well as advice regarding exercise, energy conservation, diet, relaxation, diversion and sleep-enhancement techniques as part of a broad package of interventions aimed at combating fatigue during chemotherapy. They found that patients tended to find the preparatory information about fatigue to be helpful, however the advice regarding strategies for management to be neither helpful nor unhelpful. This has important implications for occupational therapists when considering the timing of advice regarding fatigue management strategies for people with cancer. Clearly there is a need to balance the delivery of information and advice so that it occurs at a time that it is needed but prior to the stage at which the patient is too cognitively fatigued to take new information on board. Patients undergoing different treatment regimes may require information regarding fatigue to be provided at different times. For example, a patient receiving chemotherapy may benefit from information regarding fatigue prior to each cycle, however those having radiotherapy may gain more from a series of opportunities to discuss fatigue through the course of their treatment (Reuille, 2002). It should be noted that being informed about the potential for problems prior to commencing treatment can cause stress for patients, so care needs to be taken that information is provided in a measured and sensitive manner (Ream et al., 2003).

Consideration should be given to format and level of detail of information that is provided to patients. Ream et al. (2003) interviewed patients from the UK and Switzerland and found that both groups had received information related to fatigue in the form of one-to-one discussions with healthcare professionals, written materials, video, posters and the internet. They found that patients had mixed views on the benefits of most of these information formats but most had a preference towards having a variety of available options of take-home information used to supplement, rather than replace, discussions with healthcare professionals. They also found that many patients considered much of the advice provided regarding fatigue management strategies to be common sense and therefore patronizing, although others identified this same information as being useful (Ream et al., 2003). It is evident from this that occupational therapists need to adjust their approach to information provision depending upon factors such as each patient's education levels and emotional state (Portenoy and Itri, 1999). The use of standard take-home information packages should be adopted only to complement face-to-face, personalized education and support from the therapist.

The education of caregivers regarding cancer-related fatigue and its management is useful to promote recall of adherence to information and advice (Escalante, 2003). Additionally, it will provide a mechanism to support carers who themselves may feel isolated, exhausted, confused, frustrated and under-supported (Krishnasamy and Plant, 2004).

PHARMACOLOGICAL INTERVENTIONS

It has been recommended that the first step in managing cancer-related fatigue should be to identify and act upon any treatable causes such as anaemia, hypothyroidism, nutritional inadequacies, deconditioning, sleep disturbances or co-morbidities (e.g. pain, infection, cardiac or renal dysfunction). Following this, additional strategies should be adopted to manage residual fatigue that exists after the identifiable causes have been addressed (Portenoy and Itri, 1999; Mock et al., 2004; Wagner and Cella, 2004). Many of the initial fatigue management strategies may be pharmacological. Although occupational therapists will not be directly involved in the pharmacological treatment of medical problems that may contribute to fatigue (such as anaemia or infections), it remains important that they have an awareness of the impact that these issues can have upon their patients' fatigue levels due to the implications that this may have for their occupational therapy interventions. At present the evidence supporting any specific pharmacological interventions for fatigue management remains in its infancy. However, the use of erythropoietic agents (for anaemia), psychostimulants (to combat cognitive fatigue e.g. due to opioid administration) and low dose cortico-steroids have all been reported to benefit some groups of patients with fatigue (Mock *et al.*, 2004; Wagner and Cella, 2004). The use of selective serotonin-reuptake inhibitors in fatigue management is often recommended if depression is present (Portenoy and Itri, 1999; Curt, 2001; Escalante, 2003; Mock *et al.*, 2004), although strong evidence supporting the benefits of this intervention on patients' actual fatigue levels does not currently exist (Wagner and Cella, 2004).

GRADED ACTIVITY AND EXERCISE

Graded exercise is recognized as the management strategy for cancer-related fatigue that has the strongest evidence base. Numerous experimental design studies have demonstrated the benefits of aerobic exercise as a means of fatigue management in people with cancer (Mock *et al.*, 1994; Dimeo *et al.*, 1997; Mock *et al.*, 1997; Dimeo *et al.*, 1999; Schwartz *et al.*, 2000a; Dimeo *et al.*, 2004; Mock *et al.*, 2005). Watson and Mock (2003) summarized the findings of current research articles and concluded that for maximum benefit the exercise regime should:

- begin when patients commence adjuvant treatment and last for the duration of treatment;
- be of low to moderate intensity (50–70% maximum heart rate) and progressive, building from 15 to 30 minutes duration 3–5 times per week.
- be carefully and accurately recorded using an exercise diary.

Consideration should be given, however, to the patient's level of fitness prior to commencing treatment. Schwartz *et al.* (2000a) have suggested the use of structured, supervised exercise for less fit or inactive patients prior to the initiation of chemotherapy to promote adherence to exercise regimes at home post-treatment and thus reduce the impact and severity of fatigue.

Exercise has been found to have a positive effect upon the psychological well-being of people being treated for cancer-related fatigue (Dimeo *et al.*, 1999; Drouin *et al.*, 2005), and has been noted to change patients' perceptions of fatigue from a negative 'chemotherapy-induced' fatigue to a positive 'exercise-induced' state of fatigue (Adamsen *et al.*, 2004).

It is important to note that the majority of the research in support of exercise for fatigue management in cancer has been conducted with people with breast cancer, and there is currently little evidence supporting the use of exercise with people with advanced disease (Watson and Mock, 2003). As well as this there are potential contraindications for exercise in cancer rehabilitation such as cardiopulmonary risk factors, bony metastasis, neutropenia, low platelet counts, anaemia, fever or other treatment-related complications (Winningham, 2001; Mock *et al.*, 2004). Consideration should be given therefore to the medical and physical status of a patient or patient group before exercise is chosen as a fatigue management intervention (Mock *et al.*, 2004).

It is apparent that the vast majority of research with regard to the use of activity as a means of cancer-related fatigue management focuses on the benefits of aerobic exercise as opposed to functional activity. Although it is helpful and relatively easy to make a quantifiable measure of the initial status, type, intensity, frequency, duration and progression of graded exercise and thus produce measurable research or clinical results (Winningham, 2001), this does not mean that carefully chosen and monitored exercise in the form of purposeful activity would not yield similar benefits. Closer examination is needed with regard to the potential benefits of leisure, self-care or productivity-based activities that incorporate an aerobic component in order to examine their effect upon not just the physical but also the affective, social and cognitive elements of cancer-related fatigue. It would also be beneficial to investigate if the use of purposeful activity (e.g. leisure-based) as opposed to graded exercise has an impact upon the ongoing level of compliance with the fatigue management regime in the longer term. Occupational therapists working in cancer rehabilitation would be well placed to undertake research such as this.

ENERGY CONSERVATION

Energy conservation is defined by Barsevick as 'the deliberate planned management of one's personal energy resources in order to prevent their depletion' (2002, p. 16). Barsevick *et al.* (2002) list energy conservation approaches as including delegation, priority setting, pacing and planning. Cooper (1997) describes examples of energy conservation strategies such as:

- spreading out activities through the use of diaries and timetables;
- organizing activities that require more exertion at times when energy levels are likely to be high;
- prioritizing activities so as to avoid engaging in tasks that are unnecessary or not of value;
- ensuring regular breaks during activities so as to balance periods of activity and rest;
- considering posture and positioning of self and other items during activities (e.g. avoiding unnecessary bending);
- modifying activities (e.g. through the use of adaptive equipment or task simplification).

It is very important that occupational therapists making recommendations regarding energy conservation for their patients with fatigue do not adopt a 'recipe book approach' to its management. Suggestions of marked alterations to or the discarding of activities of high value can result in deteriorations in individuals' motivation and sense of self. Although many people with cancer benefit from encouragement to give themselves permission to discard or alter activities of little value that have become part of their daily routine, attempts to impose changes upon people are likely to result in them feeling a loss of control and therefore diminish the chances of success. Instead occupational therapists should spend time working closely with patients to develop individualized changes to activities or routines so as to maximize their acceptability. The energy conservation strategies adopted may need to be changed over time depending upon the patient's needs and circumstances at any given stage. Ideas that are formed through collaborative work with patients are more likely to be perceived as practical, meaningful and relevant and therefore prove successful.

It has been suggested that given the evidence supporting the benefits of activity and exercise in overcoming cancer-related fatigue the idea of adopting energy conservation strategies could be considered to be counter-productive. Indeed Richardson and Ream's (1997) investigation of patients receiving chemotherapy found energy conservation strategies to be of limited benefit. However, this would only be the case if people who utilize energy conservation techniques do so to minimize their overall daily activity, rather than to allow them to continue with a broader or more enjoyable range of activities that they enjoy. It is possible that the use of energy conservation techniques may facilitate people who encounter cancer-related fatigue to continue to engage in activities that are valuable to them. This may have broad motivational, emotional, social as well as physical benefits and thus improve people's fatigue experience. Investigations by Barsevick *et al.* (2002, 2004) found that patients who engaged in energy conservation activities reported fewer difficulties with fatigue than a control group, however the clinical significance of these findings has been questioned (Bennett, 2005). Energy conservation techniques are likely to have increased importance when working with people with deteriorating conditions due to advanced disease for whom a compensatory rather than rehabilitative approach to fatigue management is more appropriate. Further research investigating the impact of energy conservation techniques upon the short- and long-term experience of fatigue in people at different stages of the cancer trajectory should be a priority for occupational therapists.

STRUCTURED PSYCHOLOGICAL SUPPORT

Although the exact links between emotional distress and cancer-related fatigue remain unclear, many people who experience cancer-related fatigue also have correlating psychological symptoms such as anxiety and depression (Stone, Richardson *et al.*, 2000c; Ahlberg *et al.*, 2004; Brown, McMillan and Milroy, 2005). Given this, many patients with cancer-related fatigue may benefit from structured psychological strategies to augment other interventions (Bennett *et al.*, 2004). Ream and Stone (2004) emphasize that the choice of psychological interventions should be structured to meet the specific needs of individual patients, as not all patients will benefit from the same interventions. These strategies may include support groups, counselling, stress management training or tailored behavioural interventions (Mock *et al.*, 2004). Occupational therapy education entails the development of group management skills as well as skills in counselling with regard to stress and anxiety management. As a result occupational therapists can make an important contribution to the provision of structured psychological support for people experiencing problems with cancer-related fatigue through the use of strategies such as those described above.

One of the simplest, most effective but unfortunately often overlooked psychological support strategies to assist with the management of cancer-related fatigue involves taking time to listen to patients' experiences and concerns (Krishnasamy, 1997). Although educating people with cancer about fatigue and strategies to manage it is valuable, it is vital that communication about the impact of fatigue upon the person with cancer is not all therapist led. Ream *et al.* (2002) found that the people with cancer-related fatigue drew great benefit from having healthcare professionals spend time with them to listen to their experiences and provide them with support. Krishnasamy (1997, p. 131) emphasized the importance of people with advanced cancer and their carers being provided with opportunities and support to explore the existential meaning of their fatigue as an essential element in addressing the isolation and distress that it can cause. Occupational therapists can assist people affected by cancer-related fatigue who wish to communicate their thoughts and feelings about the symptom either through open discussion, or if appropriate, through the use of alternative media for expression such as the use of narratives, art or poetry.

RELAXATION AND STRUCTURED SLEEP

Sleep quality rather than quantity appears to be an important factor affecting fatigue levels of people with cancer (Ahlberg *et al.*, 2003). Although literature concerning the effectiveness of sleep intervention programmes in managing cancer-related fatigue is currently scarce, initial evaluations and feasibility studies have suggested that behavioural techniques to improve sleep patterns may help with this problem (Davidson *et al.*, 2001; Berger *et al.*, 2003). Occupational therapists should investigate the daily routines and sleep patterns of their patients presenting with cancer-related fatigue to examine the potential impact that this may be having upon their fatigue levels. Winningham (2001) recommends that patients are advised to maintain a schedule of sleeping and waking times by avoiding napping during the day time, leaving curtains open so that the sunlight awakens them in the morning, not returning to bed after getting up, avoiding 'sleeping in' on days off, and avoiding engaging in activity or eating and drinking anything in the night time that may delay sleep (e.g. heavy food or caffeine). Other suggested strategies for improving sleep in people with cancer include taking a hot bath before bed, drinking a warm glass of milk prior to bed (Escalante, 2003), and having a conducive environment for sleep (e.g. dark, quiet and comfortable or the presence of security items such as toys and blankets for children: Mock et al., 2004).

There is currently very little published research demonstrating the specific benefits of relaxation as a strategy for the management of cancer-related fatigue. Luebbert, Dahme and Hasenbring (2001) conducted a meta-analysis of the effectiveness of relaxation training in reducing treatment-related symptoms in acute non-surgical cancer patients and found no evidence of relaxation reducing fatigue levels. More recently however, Dimeo et al. (2004) compared patients post-surgically who were engaged in progressive relaxation training three times per week with those involved in an aerobic exercise programme five times per week and found that both groups made similar improvements with regard to their fatigue levels. In addition to this, the exercise group made greater improvements with regard to their exercise tolerance while the relaxation group experienced a greater reduction in pain. These findings may prove beneficial in indicating the potential benefits of relaxation in managing fatigue as well as the symptoms (such as pain) associated with fatigue in symptom clusters. It should be noted, however, that there was no control group in this particular study, and therefore the results should be interpreted with caution. Further research of the effect of different relaxation techniques on ameliorating cancer fatigue would be beneficial. Due to their skills in relaxation therapy, occupational therapists working in cancer care would be well equipped to carry out such research.

COGNITIVE REHABILITATION

Many people with cancer-related fatigue experience ongoing problems with cognitive deficits. Even if cognitive impairment is mild it can still impact on people's ability to care for themselves, to maintain or resume their previous employment, or to manage their personal relationships. Furthermore, cognitive dysfunction can impair people's ability to take on and process new information about their condition and treatment, thus compromising their ability to be involved in treatment-related decisions, adhere with treatment or therapy regimes and cope with change or loss (Cimprich and Ronis, 2003). People with cancer-related fatigue often experience difficulties with multi-tasking, short-term memory, organizational skills and word finding (Winningham,

2001). Occupational therapists have a valuable role to play in helping patients to overcome cognitive difficulties. Therapeutic activities aimed specifically at improving the cognitive components of attention, short-term memory, executive functioning and problem solving should all be considered for patients with difficulties in this area. These activities should be coupled with a broader goal specific to the patient's circumstances (e.g. independence with personal care tasks, graded return to work, or a resumption of previous leisure pursuits).

Cimprich and Ronis (2003) investigated the benefits of easy to perform, low energy attention restoring activities in natural environments (e.g. bird watching, walking or sitting in parks and gardens) in improving the capacity for attention of women newly diagnosed with breast cancer. They found that the act of being removed from an environment with high demands for mental effort into a relaxing natural environment of interest and relevance to the patient can significantly assist in the prevention and rehabilitation of difficulties with attention. Engaging people in carefully chosen therapeutic activities in appropriate environments is at the core of occupational therapy philosophy. Involvement in restorative activities such as those described to ameliorate cognitive fatigue in people with cancer should be a priority for occupational therapists working in oncology and palliative care.

In the case of assisting people to return to their work, vocational advice, workplace modifications (e.g. the development of an environment with fewer distractions or the adoption of flexible working hours) or retraining may be valuable interventions (Meyers, 2004). Occupational therapists can facilitate patients' return to work by advising them and their employers about such possible changes to tasks or the environment to assist in the management of cognitive (or general) fatigue.

SUMMARY

Cancer-related fatigue is a highly distressing symptom of cancer and its treatment that is experienced by a very large proportion of people with cancer. Occupational therapists have a unique and valuable role to play in assisting their patients to manage this symptom. For interventions to be successful a holistic view of cancer-related fatigue is essential encompassing its physical, affective, cognitive and temporal dimensions.

When screening for and assessing cancer-related fatigue occupational therapists should take into account not just the incidence of cancer-related fatigue, but also its severity, the level of distress that it causes, its meaning to the patient and its impact upon his or her daily living. Management approaches should be chosen collaboratively with the patient and personalized depending upon the individual's prognosis, medical condition or personal goals and aspirations. Depending upon individual patients' needs, interventions may be based on a rehabilitative, educative, cognitive-behavioural, psychodynamic or compensatory approach or a combination of the above.

Given the relatively new focus upon cancer-related fatigue numerous gaps in evidence still exist regarding best practice in managing the symptom. Occupational therapists have the potential to make a valuable contribution to the development of and improved understanding of the management of fatigue by engaging in and publishing well designed research relevant to their role. Given the potentially different aetiologies and patterns of fatigue experienced by people depending upon their diagnoses or the treatment they receive, attempts should be made to investigate the benefits of particular occupational therapy interventions for specific patient groups. The development and refinement of this evidence base should be a priority for occupational therapists working in cancer rehabilitation as it will ensure that the most appropriate interventions are received by people experiencing cancer-related fatigue as well as help to reinforce the importance of occupational therapy within fatigue management in cancer. This will be of benefit to people with cancer and their carers, the health service and the profession of occupational therapy.

ACTION POINTS

1. Outline the key questions an occupational therapist would use in an initial assessment with a fatigued patient, bearing in mind the burden of the assessment on the already fatigued individual.
2. Identify a case study and focus on the daily requirements of a fatigued individual and how the occupational therapy programme could be graded to help that individual cope with fatigue.
3. Explore the psychological impact of fatigue and how this can be explained to the fatigued individual and those involved in his/her care.

REFERENCES

Adamsen, L., Midtgaard, J., Roerth, M., Andersen, C., Quist, M. and Moeller, T. (2004) Transforming the nature of fatigue through exercise: Qualitative findings from a multi-dimensional exercise programme in cancer patients undergoing chemotherapy. *European Journal of Cancer Care*, **13**(4), 362–70.

Ahlberg, K., Ekman, T., Gaston-Johansson, F. and Mock, V. (2003) Assessment and management of cancer-related fatigue in adults. *The Lancet*, **362**(9384), 640–66.

Ahlberg, K., Ekman, T., Wallgreen, A. and Gaston-Johansson, F. (2004) Fatigue, psychological distress, coping and quality of life in patients with uterine cancer. *Journal of Advanced Nursing*, **45**(2), 205–13.

Barsevick, A. M. (2002) Energy conservation and cancer-related fatigue. *Rehabilitation Oncology*, **20**(3), 14–18.

Barsevick, A. M., Whitmer, K., Sweeny, C. and Nail, L. M. (2002) A pilot study examining energy conservation for cancer treatment-related fatigue. *Cancer Nursing*, **25**(5), 333–41.

Barsevick, A. M., Dudley, W., Beck, S., Sweeney, C., Whitmer, K. and Nail, L. (2004) A randomized clinical trial of energy conservation for patients with cancer-related fatigue. *Cancer*, **100**(6), 1302–10.

Bennett, B., Goldstein, D., Lloyd, A., Davenport, T. and Hickie, I. (2004) Fatigue and psychological distress – exploring the relationship in women treated for breast cancer. *European Journal of Cancer*, **40**(11), 1689–95.

Bennett, S. (2005) Commentary – An energy conservation program for people with cancer produced small changes in fatigue. *Australian Occupational Therapy Journal*, **52**(1), 90–1.

Berger, A. M. (1998) Patterns of fatigue and activity and rest during adjuvant breast cancer chemotherapy. *Oncology Nursing Forum*, **25**(1), 51–62.

Berger, A. M., VonEssen, S., Kuhn, B., Piper, B. F., Farr, L., Agrawal, S., Lynch, J. C. and Higginbotham, P. (2003) Adherence, sleep and fatigue outcomes after adjuvant breast cancer chemotherapy: Results of a feasibility intervention study. *Oncology Nursing Forum*, **30**(3), 513–22.

Borthwick, D., Knowles, G., McNamara, S., O'Dea, R. and Stroner, P. (2003) Assessing fatigue and self-care strategies in patients receiving radiotherapy for non-small cell lung cancer. *European Journal of Oncology Nursing*, **7**(4), 231–41.

Brown, D. J. F., McMillan, D. C. and Milroy, R. (2005) The correlation between fatigue, physical function, the systemic inflammatory response, and psychological distress in patients with advanced lung cancer. *Cancer*, **103**(2), 377–82.

Cimprich, B. and Ronis, D. L. (2001) Attention and symptom distress in women with and without breast cancer. *Nursing Research*, **50**(2), 86–94.

Cimprich, B. and Ronis, D. L. (2003) An environmental intervention to restore attention in women with newly diagnosed breast cancer. *Cancer Nursing*, **26**(4), 284–92.

Cooley, M. E., Short, T. H. and Moriarty, H. J. (2003) Symptom prevalence, distress, and change over time in adults receiving treatment for lung cancer. *Psycho-oncology*, **12**(7), 694–708.

Cooper, J. (1997) *Occupational Therapy in Oncology and Palliative Care*, Whurr, London.

Curt, G. A. (2001) Fatigue in cancer. *British Medical Journal*, **322**(7302), 1560.

Curt, G. A., Breitbart, W., Cella, D., Gropman, J. E., Horning, S. J., Itri, L. M. *et al.* (2000) Impact of cancer-related fatigue on the lives of patients: New findings from the fatigue coalition. *Oncologist*, **5**(5), 353–60.

Davidson, J. R., Waisberg, J. L., Brundage, M. D. and MacLean, A. W. (2001) Non-pharmacological group treatment of insomnia: A preliminary study with cancer survivors. *Psycho-oncology*, **10**(5), 389–97.

de Jong, N., Courtens, A. M., Abu-Saad, H. H. and Schouten, H. C. (2002) Fatigue in patients with breast cancer receiving adjuvant chemotherapy: A review of the literature. *Cancer Nursing*, **25**(4), 283–97.

Dimeo, F. C., Stielglitz, R. D., Novelli-Fischer, U., Fetscher, S. and Keul, J. (1999) Effects of physical activity on the fatigue and psychological status of patients during chemotherapy. *Cancer*, **85**(10), 2273–77.

Dimeo, F. C., Thomas, F., Raabe-Menssen, C., Propper, F. and Mathias, M. (2004) Effect of aerobic exercise and relaxation training on fatigue and physical performance of cancer patients after surgery. A randomised controlled trial. *Supportive Care in Cancer*, **12**(11), 774–9.

Dimeo, F. C., Tilmann, M. H., Bertz, H., Kanz, L., Mertelsmann, R. and Keul, J. (1997) Aerobic exercise in the rehabilitation of cancer patients after high dose chemotherapy and autologous peripheral stem cell transplantation. *Cancer*, **79**(9), 1717–22.

Dodd, M. J., Miaskowski, C. and Paul, S. M. (2001) Symptom clusters and their effect on the functional status of patients with cancer. *Oncology Nursing Forum*, **28**(3), 465–70.

Donnelly, S. (1998) Patient management strategies for interferon alfa-2b as adjuvant therapy of high-risk melanoma. *Oncology Nursing Forum*, **25**(5), 921–7.

Drouin, J. S., Armstrong, H., Krause, S., Orr, J., Birk, T. J., Hryniuk, W. et al. (2005) Effects of aerobic exercise training on peak aerobic capacity, fatigue and psychological factors during radiation for breast cancer. *Rehabilitation Oncology*, **23**(1), 11–17.

Escalante, C. (2003) Treatment of cancer-related fatigue: An update. *Supportive Care in Cancer*, **11**, 79–83.

Figlin, R., Belldegrun, A., Moldawer, N., Zeffren, J. and de Kernion, J. (1992) Concomitant administration of recombinant human interleukin-2 and recombinant alfa-2A: An active outpatient regime in metastatic renal cell carcinoma. *Journal of Clinical Oncology*, **10**, 414–21.

Fu, M. R., Anderson, C. M., McDaniel, R. and Armer, J. (2002) Patient's perceptions of fatigue in response to biochemotherapy for metastatic melanoma: A preliminary study. *Oncology Nursing Forum*, **29**(6), 961–6.

Galloway, S. C. and Graydon, J. E. (1996) Uncertainty, symptom distress and information needs after surgery for cancer of the colon. *Cancer Nursing*, **19**(2), 112–17.

Given, C., Given, B., Azzouz, F., Kozachik, S. and Stommel, M. (2001) Predictors of pain and fatigue in the year following diagnosis among elderly cancer patients. *Journal of Pain and Symptom Management*, **21**(6), 456–66.

Horng-Shiuann, W. and McSweeny, M. (2004) The assessment and measurement of fatigue in people with cancer, in *Fatigue in Cancer* (eds J. Armes, M. Krishnasamy and I. Higginson), Oxford University Press, Oxford.

Jacobsen, P. B., Hann, D. M., Azzarello, L. M., Horton, J., Balducci, L. and Lyman, G. H. (1999) Fatigue in women receiving adjuvant chemotherapy for breast cancer: Characteristics, course and correlates. *Journal of Pain and Symptom Management*, **18**(4), 233–42.

Jereczek-Fossa, B. A., Marsiglia H. R. and Orecchia, R. (2002) Radiotherapy-related fatigue. *Critical Reviews in Oncology/Hematology*, **41**(3), 317–25.

Kearney, N., Miller, M., Weir-Hughes, D., Sermeus, W., Hoy, D., Gibson, F. *et al.* (2004) *Wisecare+ Final Report*. Cancer Care Research Centre and The Royal Marsden NHS Foundation Trust, London.

Krishnasamy, M. (1997) Exploring the nature and impact of fatigue in advanced cancer. *International Journal of Palliative Nursing*, **3**(3), 126–31.

Krishnasamy, M. (2004) Commentary – Assessing fatigue and self-care strategies in patients receiving radiotherapy for non-small cell lung cancer, by D. Borthwick, G. Knowles, S. McNamara, R. O'Dea, P. Stroner. *European Journal of Oncology Nursing*, 8, 83–4.

Krishnasamy, M. and Plant, H. (2004) Carers, caring, and cancer-related fatigue, in *Fatigue in Cancer* (eds J. Armes, M. Krishnasamy and I. Higginson), Oxford University Press, Oxford.

Luebbert, K., Dahme, B. and Hasenbring, M. (2001) The effectiveness of relaxation training in reducing treatment-related symptoms and improving emotional adjustment in acute non-surgical cancer treatment: A meta analytic review. *Psycho-oncology*, **10**(6), 490–502.

Madhusudan, S., Foster, M., Muthuramalingam, S. R., Braybrooke, J. P., Wilner, S., Kaur, K. et al. (2004) A phase II study of etanercept (enbrel), a tumor necrosis factor α inhibitor in patients with metastatic breast cancer. *Clinical Cancer Research*, **10**(19), 6528–34.

Meyers, C. A. (2004) Mental fatigue and cognitive dysfunction, in *Fatigue in Cancer* (eds J. Armes, M. Krishnasamy and I. Higginson), Oxford University Press, Oxford.

Mock, V., Atkinson, A., Barsevick, A., Cella, D., Cimprich, B., Cleeland, C. et al., for the National Comprehensive Cancer Network Cancer-related Fatigue Panel (2004) *NCCN Clinical Practice Guidelines in Oncology – Cancer-related Fatigue, Version 1*. National Comprehensive Cancer Network © NCCN 2004. http://www.nccn.org (Accessed 7.8.04)

Mock, V., Barton Burke, M., Sheehan, P., Creaton, E. M., Winningham, M. L., McKenney-Tedder, S. et al. (1994) A nursing rehabilitation program for women with breast cancer receiving adjuvant chemotherapy. *Oncology Nursing Forum*, **21**(5), 899–908.

Mock, V., Hassey Dow, K., Meares, C. J., Grimm, P. M., Dienemann, J. A., Haisfield-Wolfe, M. E. et al. (1997) Effects of exercise on fatigue, physical functioning, and emotional distress during radiation therapy for breast cancer. *Oncology Nursing Forum*, **24**(6), 991–1000.

Mock, V., Frangakis, C., Davidson, N. E., Ropka, M. E., Pickett, M., Poniatowski, B. et al. (2005) Exercise manages fatigue during breast cancer treatment: A randomized controlled trial. *Psycho-oncology*, **14**(6), 464–77.

Okuyama, T., Tanaka, K., Akechi, T., Kugaya, A., Okamura, H., Nishiwaki, Y. et al. (2001) Fatigue in ambulatory patients with advanced lung cancer: Prevalence, correlated factors and screening. *Journal of Pain and Symptom Management*, **22**(1), 554–64.

Piper, B. F. (2004) Measuring fatigue. *Instruments for Clinical Health-Care Research*, 3rd edn (eds M. Frank-Stromborg and S. J. Olsen), Jones and Bartlett Publishers, Ontario.

Porock, D. and Juenger, J. A. (2004) Just go with the flow: A qualitative study of fatigue in biotherapy. *European Journal of Cancer Care*, **13**(4), 356–61.

Portenoy, R. and Itri, L. M. (1999) Cancer-related fatigue: Guidelines for evaluation and management. *The Oncologist*, **4**(1), 1–10.

Ream, E., Browne, N., Glaus, A., Knipping, C. and Frei, I. A. (2003) Quality and efficacy of educational materials on cancer-related fatigue: Views of patients from two European countries. *European Journal of Oncology Nursing*, **7**(2), 99–109.

Ream, E. and Richardson, A. (1996) Fatigue: A concept analysis. *International Journal of Nursing Studies*, **33**(5), 519–29.

Ream, E., Richardson, A. and Alexander-Dann, C. (2002) Facilitating patients' coping with fatigue during chemotherapy – pilot outomes. *Cancer Nursing*, **25**(4), 300–8.

Ream, E. and Stone, P. (2004) Clinical interventions for fatigue, in *Fatigue in Cancer* (eds J. Armes, M. Krishnasamy and M. Higginson), Oxford University Press, Oxford.

Reuille, K. M. (2002) Using self-regulation theory to develop an intervention for cancer-related fatigue. *Clinical Nurse Specialist*, **16**(6), 312–19.

Richardson, A. (1994) The health diary: An example of its use as a data collection method. *Journal of Advanced Nursing*, **19**, 782–91.

Richardson, A. (1998) Measuring fatigue in patients with cancer. *Supportive Care in Cancer*, **6**(2), 94–100.

Richardson, A. (2004) A critical appraisal of the factors associated with fatigue, in *Fatigue in Cancer* (eds J. Armes, M. Krishnasamy and M. Higginson), Oxford University Press, Oxford.

Richardson, A. and Ream, E. (1996) Fatigue in patients receiving chemotherapy for advanced cancer. *International Journal of Palliative Nursing*, **2**(4), 199–204.

Richardson, A. and Ream, E. (1997) Self-care behaviours initiated by chemotherapy patients in response to fatigue. *International Journal of Nursing Studies*, **34**(1), 35–43.

Richardson, A. and Ream, E. (1998) Recent progress in understanding cancer-related fatigue. *International Journal of Palliative Nursing*, **4**(4), 192–8.

Richardson, A., Ream, E. and Wilson-Barnett, J. (1998) Fatigue in patients receiving chemotherapy: Patterns of change. *Cancer Nursing*, **21**(3), 195.

Ruckdeschel, J. C. (2005) Fatigue is becoming an exhausting problem. *Cancer*, **103**(2), 213–15.

Schwartz, A. L., Mori, M., Gao, R., Nail, L. M. and King, M. E. (2000a) Exercise reduces daily fatigue in women with breast cancer receiving chemotherapy. *Medicine and Science in Sports and Exercise*, **33**(5), 718–23.

Schwartz, A. L., Nail, L. M., Chen, S., Meek, P., Barsevick, A. M., King, M. E. *et al.* (2000b) Fatigue patterns observed in patients receiving chemotherapy and radiotherapy. *Cancer Investigation*, **18**(1), 11–19.

Servaes, P., Verhagen, C. and Bleijenberg, G. (2002) Fatigue in cancer patients during and after treatment: Prevalence, correlates and interventions. *European Journal of Cancer*, **38**(1), 27–43.

Stone, P., Hardy, J., Huddart, R., A'Hern, R. and Richards, M. (2000a) Fatigue in patients with prostate cancer receiving hormone therapy. *European Journal of Cancer*, **36**(9), 1134–41.

Stone, P., Richards, M., A'Hern, R. and Hardy, J. (2000b) A study to investigate the prevalence, severity and correlates of fatigue among patients with cancer in comparison with a control group of volunteers without cancer. *Annals of Oncology*, **11**(5), 561–7.

Stone, P., Richardson, A., Ream, E., Smith, A. G., Kerr, D. J. and Kearney, N. (2000c) Cancer-related fatigue: Inevitable, unimportant and untreatable? Results of a multi-centre patient survey. *Annals of Oncology*, **11**(8), 971–5.

Volgelzang, N. J., Breitbart, W., Cella, D., Curt, G. A., Groopman, J. E., Horning, S. J. *et al.* (1997) Patient, caregiver, and oncologist perceptions of cancer-related fatigue: Results of a tri-part assessment survey. *Seminars in Haematology*, **34**(3 Suppl 2), 4–12.

Wagner, L. I. and Cella, D. (2004) Fatigue and cancer: Causes, prevalence and treatment approaches. *British Journal of Cancer*, **91**(5), 822–8.

Watson, T. and Mock, V. (2003) Exercise and cancer-related fatigue: A review of the literature. *Rehabilitation Oncology*, **21**(1), 23–32.

Winningham, M. L. (2001) Strategies for managing cancer-related fatigue syndrome: A rehabilitation approach. *Cancer*, **92**(4 Suppl), 988–97.

Woo, B., Dibble, S. L., Piper, B. F., Keating, S. B. and Weiss, M. C. (1998) Differences in fatigue by treatment methods in women with breast cancer. *Oncology Nursing Forum*, **25**(5), 915–20.

7 Client-centred Approach of Occupational Therapy Programme – Case Study

GEMMA LINDSELL

PERSONAL, FAMILY, SOCIAL AND MEDICAL HISTORY

Mrs X is a 55-year-old woman, with two children: a son aged 27 years, and a daughter aged 23 years. Mrs X is married, but has been estranged from her husband for 4 years; he still shares the family home. Prior to this admission, Mrs X worked as a computer analyst, and would like to return to this line of work in the future. Mrs X has a family history of breast cancer, including her mother and two aunts.

Twelve years prior to amputation, Mrs X had undergone two courses of chemotherapy followed by radiotherapy for cancer of her left breast. These therapies failed to produce any reduction in the size of the tumour, so Mrs X underwent a modified radical left-sided mastectomy, which included excision of the lymph nodes of the left axilla. Sixteen of the 27 nodes excised were subsequently found to be cancerous. Two years after her mastectomy, Mrs X had reconstructive surgery. Last year, she underwent further plastic surgery to create a nipple for the reconstructed breast, which gave an 'excellent cosmetic result'.

Mrs X had returned to work after her mastectomy, continued to take tamoxifen (which she would need to take for five years), and received 6-monthly mammograms of her right breast. There was no evidence of recurrent cancer until January of this year, when she presented to her GP with a large, necrotic lesion in her left axilla. After an MRI (magnetic resonance imaging) scan and a biopsy of the lesion, Mrs X was diagnosed with a radiation-induced angiosarcoma of the left axilla.

Sarcomas are malignant lesions occurring in the soft tissues and bone (Cooper, 1997). The soft tissues are those that connect, support and surround anatomic structures. Angiosarcomas are rare, highly malignant tumours occurring in the vascular endothelium (Souhami and Tobias, 1995), usually arising in the skin, subcutaneous tissues and glandular sites, such as the breast and thyroid.

Occupational Therapy in Oncology and Palliative Care. Edited by J. Cooper
© 2006 John Wiley & Sons Ltd

Mrs X received two courses of chemotherapy, to which the tumour failed to respond. Surgical exploration of the area revealed that the tumour was quite advanced, and had extended to and involved the brachial plexus. Excision of the tumour would not be possible, so Mrs X underwent a left forequarter amputation, with curative intent. This involved the complete removal of the left arm, along with the scapula and clavicle. Amputation commonly results in the 'phantom limb phenomenon', the individual's awareness of residual pain or sensation in the absent limb. Mrs X experienced a painful burning sensation in her absent limb, a phenomenon that lasts for years for some patients, possibly due to the division of major nerves at the stump which provides 'inappropriate sensory stimuli for the central nervous system' (Colburn and Ibbotson, 1996).

OCCUPATIONAL THERAPY
ASSESSMENT METHODS

Referral was made to occupational therapy for functional assessment and rehabilitation following a left-sided (non-dominant) forequarter amputation. No formal standardized assessments were used as part of occupational therapy intervention with Mrs X. However, examples of standardized assessments that may have been relevant to use are the Assessment of Motor and Process Skills (AMPS) (Neistadt, 2000) and the Rehabilitation Institute of Chicago (RIC) Functional Assessment Scale (Culler, 1993). AMPS examines motor and process skills required in activities of daily living (ADLs) task performance. It would have been appropriate for use with Mrs X as it assesses skills including posture, mobility and strength and also the adaptive capacities needed to carry out tasks. The RIC Functional Assessment Scale also assesses physically disabled patients' ability to carry out ADL tasks and recognizes that patients have varied lifestyles and responsibilities, and one of its aims is to capture these differences in lifestyle so that they can be incorporated into evaluation, goal setting, and treatment planning.

Mrs X's functional abilities were assessed using the following methods:

1. initial interview: an informal discussion with Mrs X in order to gain an insight into her previous level of functioning, details of her home environment, leisure interests, and her perception of any anticipated functional difficulties that may follow discharge from hospital;
2. assessment of transfers, i.e. bed, bath, chair and toilet;
3. domestic activities of daily living assessment, i.e. making a hot drink; meal preparation, which is discussed in the activity analysis;

4. home visit;
5. liaison with physiotherapist;
6. liaison with ward staff.

RESULTS AND IDENTIFICATION OF STRENGTHS AND PROBLEMS

The occupational therapy department does not follow one particular theoretical model, but is influenced by the Canadian Occupational Performance Measure (COPM) (Sumsion, 1999). The COPM divides occupation into three main areas (Sumsion, 1999):

- self-care
- productivity
- leisure.

The model also focuses on three components of occupational performance:

- affective
- physical
- cognitive.

According to the COPM, the client's environment is also an important aspect to consider, as it can be either enabling or constraining (Law *et al.*, 1997). All of these areas were considered when identifying Mrs X's functional strengths and problems, using the assessment methods mentioned earlier. Consistent with the holistic nature of the COPM, the social and psychological aspects of Mrs X's disability were considered as well as issues relating to functional ability. These are important considerations, as these aspects can impact on how clients adapt to their disability, as can be seen in Table 7.1.

PSYCHOSOCIAL ISSUES

Cancer is perceived as a very threatening disease, and has been described as one of our culture's taboo subjects (Calman and Hine, 1995). 30–47% of cancer patients experience psychological distress following diagnosis (Zabalegui, 1999). The word 'cancer' strikes fear into people (Sarafino, 1998); it is a disease with a reputation of almost mythological proportions (Greaves, 2000). Scambler (1997) stated, 'If in the nineteenth century tuberculosis stood out as the disease arousing the most dread and repulsion, cancer is its twentieth century equivalent.' Much of the fear evoked by cancer is in relation to fear of losses it can provoke. Among these are loss of:

Table 7.1 Adapting to disability

Occupational performance area	Strengths identified	Problems identified
	(Assessment methods in brackets)	
Self-care	• Mrs X can independently attend to most of her self-care needs (1)	• Mrs X has difficulty doing up buttons (1) • Mrs X is unable to tie shoelaces with one hand (1) • Mrs X has impaired balance following her amputation, which reduces her safety and independence in bath transfers (1,2,3,6)
Productivity	• Mrs X is well-motivated to return to her work role (1)	• Mrs X wishes to return to her premorbid role of meal-provider for her children (1) • Mrs X may have difficulty using a computer with one hand at work (1)
Leisure	• Mrs X reports that she wishes to become involved in an exercise group for amputees (1)	
Affective		• Mrs X's confidence and self-esteem are reduced following body image change (1,6)
Physical	• Mrs X can perform all transfers with minimal assistance to ensure safety (e.g. uses grab rails in bath transfers) (2)	• Mrs X's balance is impaired by amputation (2,3,5,6) • Mrs X experiences 'phantom pain' in her absent limb (1,5,6)
Cognitive	• Mrs X appears to have no problems in this area (1,2,3,4,5,6)	
Environment	• Mrs X has a strong and supportive social environment (1,6)	• Mrs X's home environment requires modification to facilitate maximum independence and safety (1,5)

- physical strength and well-being
- independence
- roles
- interpersonal relationships
- sexual function
- life expectancy
- control
- mental integrity.

(Barraclough, 1994)

Cancer patients usually employ a combination of the following coping strategies in order to manage their stressors:

- seeking and using social support (this involves establishing connections with individuals who can offer informational, tangible or emotional support);
- escape-avoidance (this involves the avoidance of stressors through fantasy or wishful thinking);
- distancing (this involves dealing objectively with the stressor by minimizing its significance);
- focusing on the positive (this involves taking a constructive attitude and the use of positive thinking).

(Zabalegui, 1999)

Mrs X employed the use of the last of these strategies in dealing with her cancer and also her subsequent forequarter amputation. This strategy includes the individual 'finding new faith, rediscovering what is good in life, and changing or growing as a person in a good way' (Zabalegui, 1999). She resolved to join an exercise group for amputees on her discharge from hospital, illustrating a willingness to initiate a new leisure interest and seeking of network support to provide a feeling of membership within a group (Sarafino, 1998). It is such constructive actions that are associated with improved outcomes; individuals who display this tend to adapt better than those who feel helpless, believing there is nothing they can do to improve their situation (Faulkner and Maguire, 1994). Mrs X can be said to demonstrate a sense of self-efficacy in her motivation to change an aspect of her health behaviour (by taking up regular exercise) and thereby enhance her health (Taylor, 1995).

Mrs X's decision to start practising regular physical exercise is constructive in itself: it has both psychological and physical benefits (Maguire and Parkes, 1998). Exercise can help increase self-esteem and reduce stress (Taylor, 1995; Maguire and Parkes, 1998). Also, exercise has been shown to increase endogenous opioids in the body, thus being effective in reducing pain (Taylor, 1995).

Amputation can have profound psychological effects on the individual (Colburn and Ibbotson, 1992). The experience of a newly acquired disability can produce cyclic feelings of 'disbelief, denial, anger, panic, self-devaluation and guilt, alternating with feelings of relief and exultation' (Yerxa, 1996). Commonly, the individual also experiences a sense of loss and a phase of mourning (Yerxa, 1996) similar to that experienced by the bereaved (Maguire and Parkes, 1998).

It has been found that individuals who repress or avoid these feelings of grief following limb loss tend to experience more phantom limb pain than other amputees (Maguire and Parkes, 1998). It has been suggested that the phantom phenomena can result, in part, from the individual's need to compensate for the void in their body image (Guex, 1994). Encouraging patients to confront their loss and grief can reduce their experience of phantom pain (Fisher and Hanspal, 1998). The use of guided imagery (to re-focus patients' attention) has also been found to be beneficial (Price, 2000).

Not only has Mrs X experienced body image alteration through her amputation, but also through her hair loss (induced by chemotherapy). Body image change, such as hair loss, can also lead to decreased self-esteem, grief and depression (Maguire and Parkes, 1998). Mrs X's previous mastectomy is likely to have impacted upon her self-image, also, as this can generate feelings of a loss of 'wholeness' (Faulkner and Maguire, 1994) and diminished femininity: the breast is symbolic of 'womanliness, sexual attractiveness, and nurturance' (Mock, 1993).

An amputation of a body part, such as experienced by Mrs X, causes the individual to be stigmatized due to its very visible nature (Goffman, 1968). Individuals with noticeable disfigurement are discredited in our society, which holds the belief that 'physical beauty is good, and deformity bad' (Newell, 2000). Cancer can cause individuals to feel stigmatized (Faulkner and Maguire, 1994). It is fairly common for the patient to become estranged from family and friends who may distance themselves from the patient due to social awkwardness (Sarafino, 1998) and the desire to avoid confronting distressing issues (Faulkner and Maguire, 1994).

Cancer can contribute to an external locus of control (Faulkner and Maguire, 1994). Cancer patients commonly experience a sense of loss of control over their lives due to the uncertain nature of the disease's cause, course, prognosis and treatment (Lloyd and Coggles, 1990). Mrs X however, showed an internal locus of control, to some degree, in that she took responsibility for her own health by deciding to join the exercise group (Taylor, 1995).

Her cancer, and subsequent amputation, have led to the loss of Mrs X's work role, to which she intends to return as soon as she is able. Productivity is highly valued in western society (Bye, 1998), and loss of this role can lead to reduced self-worth, an alteration in self-identity, economic hardship, depression, forced inactivity and dependence (Burt and Smith, 1996). Mrs X displayed a sense of self-efficacy with regard to this issue, in her expression of her determination to return to this role (Sarafino, 1998).

Cancer has been said to 'invade' families (Parkes, 1998); it affects many lives, not just that of the patient (Maguire and Parkes, 1998). Diagnosis of cancer leads to the family experience of anticipatory grieving (Lloyd and Coggles, 1990). It invariably contributes to family tensions, as roles and responsibilities are redistributed. It can be especially difficult for children whose parent has cancer; they may react with feelings of fear, anger, a sense of having been cheated, or irrational guilt that they may have caused the disease (Cancerlink, 2001). It is also very difficult for them to cope with changes in usual routines, leading to insecurity and resentment. Mrs X's children are currently undergoing counselling to help them come to terms with their mother's diagnosis.

Mrs X is estranged from her husband, from whom she is separated but with whom she still lives. It has been found that cancer can strengthen and enhance some relationships (Barraclough, 1994); however, it has been noted that it can increase the strain on problematic relationships (Faulkner and Maguire, 1994). Marriage has been proven to be an important source of social and emotional support for those facing stressful life events; mortality rates for married people are lower than those for single people. The lack of a relationship in which mutual confidences are shared is related to decreased quality of life and reduced ability to cope with stressful life events such as cancer (Vachon, 1998).

Mrs X would appear to have a fairly wide and supportive social network of friends. This would suggest that she is more likely to maintain physical and psychological health than an individual with few social contacts, as a correlation has been identified between social support and well-being.

PROFESSIONAL ISSUES

Although the occupational therapy approach in this case study did not utilize any one theoretical model to guide intervention, a rehabilitative and adaptive approach was used and was influenced by the following model and frame of reference. The Canadian Occupational Performance Measure (COPM) influences interventions, and this model is discussed here due to its relevance to Mrs X and its appropriateness for use within an oncology setting.

The COPM describes a dynamic interaction between individuals, their occupations and roles, and the environments within which they perform them (Law et al., 1997). Affective, cognitive, physical and spiritual aspects are interconnected with the occupational performance areas (self-care, productivity and leisure) and also with the client's various environments.

The model emphasizes the central importance of the individual, which is reflected in the model's alliance with client-centred practice (Law et al., 1997).

Central to the individual, the model recognizes the element of spirituality, which is viewed as the essence of the client's truest self, and which is expressed through the performance of occupations. In this way, the model is holistic, regarding individuals as a whole, including their physical, social, psychological and cultural needs (Law *et al.*, 1994). This was important with regard to Mrs X: the occupational therapist recognized the necessity to address the psychosocial aspects of her disability, as well as physical or functional implications.

Sumsion (1999) discusses how gaining an understanding of the client's essence of himself actually helps in planning an individualized treatment plan. Sumsion (1999) also suggests that acknowledging their spirituality and what is important to the clients is also a way of acknowledging the clients' inner strength. In order to understand the clients' personal meaning and experiences, it is the occupational therapist's role to listen to the client's narrative (Hammell, 1998).

Traditionally, occupational therapy intervention has focused on the physical environment (Sumsion, 1999). However, the COPM recognizes the influence that social, cultural and institutional environments also have upon the client's occupational performance (Law *et al.*, 1997). In the case of Mrs X, the intervention plan needs to encompass not only her physical environment, but also her social environment (addressing issues related to interpersonal relationships and family environment) and institutional environment (regarding accessibility to organizations and support groups, and addressing employment issues).

The rehabilitative frame of reference was used with Mrs X. This is based on the use of compensatory strategies in order to minimize functional limitation (Foster, 1992). These strategies involve the use of adaptive devices, modification of the environment, and adapted procedures (Dutton, 1995; Bain, 1998) to facilitate compensation in the face of deficits that cannot be remediated (Dutton, 1995). All three strategies were used in interventions with Mrs X.

Consistent with the COPM, the rehabilitative frame of reference focuses on clients' functional abilities in the areas of self-care, productivity and leisure (Seidel, 1998). It emphasizes the importance of clients' competency in daily activities; practise of activities of daily living is a significant aspect of the intervention programme.

Like the COPM, which acknowledges every individual's potential to change (Law *et al.*, 1997), the rehabilitative frame of reference embraces the individual's existing abilities (Seidel, 1998). These strengths are optimized through the application of compensatory methods in order to bring about change in the client's capacity for functional independence.

A teaching–learning process is central to this frame of reference, so that the client can learn to apply new techniques to perform occupations (Seidel, 1998). In accordance with this, Mrs X was provided with resources and also opportunities to experiment with adaptive equipment and compensatory strategies. The rehabilitative frame of reference places importance on the learning environment; treatment programmes should occur in the environment that is natural for the performance of the activities (Seidel, 1998). Consistent with this, interventions related to activities of daily living took place within the occupational therapy department kitchen and bathroom to maximize learning.

This frame of reference, like the COPM, is holistic in nature. It not only addresses functional ability, but also clients' interests, roles, resources, environments, and support systems (Seidel, 1998).

The client-centred approach was used with Mrs X, which is strongly consistent with the COMP, and also with the rehabilitative frame of reference since the individual must be at the core of rehabilitation (Baum, 1998). Through the application of this approach, the client defines the most important areas for intervention (Law *et al.*, 1995). This ensures that the intervention programme addresses goals that are meaningful to the individual (Law *et al.*, 1997), and that it is relevant to their life roles (Culler, 1998).

Respect and credence are given to the clients' perspective of their disability; the therapist recognizes that clients are the 'experts' with regard to their functional abilities (Law and Mills, 1998). This creates a relationship wherein client and therapist learn from each other's expertise.

The client-centred approach requires that the therapist and client build a therapeutic relationship based on mutual trust (Sumsion, 1999). This is essential in facilitating the teaching–learning relationship emphasized in the rehabilitative frame of reference, as it means that the client can feel confident in questioning fears and issues (Law and Mills, 1995; Sumsion, 1999).

As part of the client-centred approach, it is incumbent upon the therapist to make resources and information accessible to the clients. This enables clients to make informed choices and decisions in accordance with their needs and with regard to the desired outcomes of intervention (Law *et al.*, 1995). Throughout the intervention programme with Mrs X, there was an emphasis on provision of relevant resources and information. This encourages the client to take an active role in the occupational therapy process, promoting self-directedness and acceptance of responsibility (Yerxa, 1996). Giving clients an active role in their treatment allows them to experience a sense of mastery, independence and increased self-esteem (McColl *et al.*, 1997). The client-centred approach has been found to improve client satisfaction and also compliance with treatment (Law *et al.*, 1995). In summary, these theories were used in conjunction with one another to form a treatment plan that recognized and utilized Mrs X's strengths, and encouraged her to accept responsibility for adaptation to her disability. Interventions were concerned with empowerment and education, and incorporated goals that were relevant to her lifestyle.

OCCUPATIONAL THERAPY PROGRAMME

Intervention with Mrs X began a few days before her surgery. It is part of the occupational therapist's role to provide reassurance to clients during the pre-operative, post-operative and rehabilitation phases of care. By making contact with Mrs X before her surgery, this enabled the occupational therapist to introduce herself and begin establish a trusting, reciprocal, respectful relationship – a key element of the client-centred approach (Hammell, 1998). Another aim of making contact with the client prior to her amputation was to address any concerns related to daily living that Mrs X might be anticipating. It also reflects a holistic element to the intervention, as it encouraged Mrs X to think about and confront her fears regarding her forthcoming disability.

Mrs X was not seen again until a week after her operation. She was medically stable, and ready to begin rehabilitation. At this point, the initial assessment was carried out, in order to gain information regarding Mrs X's home situation and to re-assess Mrs X's views about any functional problems she was experiencing. This assessment highlighted the fact that Mrs X wanted to be able to continue to perform all the activities that she had carried out premorbidly; it also indicated that modifications would need to be made to Mrs X's home environment.

PRIORITIZED PROBLEM LIST

With input from the patient, a prioritized problem list was formulated (see Table 7.2), ensuring that the intervention would be pertinent to Mrs X's life roles (Culler, 1998). These priorities formed the basis of the intervention plan, which would focus on Mrs X's rehabilitation: to enable her to adapt to her new disability, and enable her to function as independently as possible in the areas of self-care, productivity and leisure. The intervention plan placed importance on Mrs X's return to her life roles, which is a core skill of occupational therapy.

GOAL OF INTERVENTION

The goal of intervention with Mrs X was to facilitate adaptation to her acquired disability and to enable her to carry out activities of daily living and to fulfil life roles.

THERAPEUTIC AIMS

The following aims were set, to facilitate achievement of the above long-term goal:

Table 7.2 Prioritized problem list

Order of prioritization	Problem	Reason for prioritization	Problem identified by client (c), therapist (t), or both (b)
1	• Mrs X wishes to be able to fulfil role of meal provider to her children	• Inability to carry out this role could lead to further family disruption • Ability to fulfil this role is important for Mrs X's self-concept • May contribute to health and well-being of children	c
2	• Mrs X's home requires modification in order to create an enabling and safe environment for discharge	• Mrs X's safety may be compromised due to impaired balance • Will facilitate greater independence	b
3	• Mrs X may experience difficulty carrying out her work role with one arm	• Return to work may be necessary for maintenance of self-esteem and stimulation • Mrs X wishes to return to her work role	c
4	• Mrs X requires minimal assistance with dressing (i.e. attending to fastenings)	• Will facilitate greater independence	b
5	• Mrs X's self-image has been affected by her amputation	• May impact on functional level • May affect maintenance of interpersonal relationships • May impact on Mrs X's adaptation to her disability	b

1. for Mrs X to be able to prepare hot meals independently, and safely;
2. for Mrs X's home to be adapted to facilitate maximum independence and safety;
3. for Mrs X to be able to manage all aspects of dressing, using compensatory techniques and adaptive equipment where necessary;
4. for Mrs X to be able to return to carry out her work role;
5. for Mrs X to acknowledge and express the psychological implications of her amputation, to facilitate adjustment to her situation.

THERAPEUTIC OBJECTIVES

Treatment objectives were agreed for each of the above aims, with a time frame of three weeks, by which time the ward's medical team anticipated that Mrs X would be ready for discharge home.

Aim 1 – objectives

- Mrs X will begin by practising hot drink preparation in the occupational therapy department kitchen.
- Mrs X will try out various items of assistive equipment in the occupational therapy department kitchen.
- Mrs X will select a suitable recipe and inform the occupational therapist of her choice, in order that the necessary ingredients can be purchased.
- Mrs X will carry out meal preparation in the occupational therapy kitchen.
- Mrs X will increase her activity tolerance from 45 minutes to 90 minutes plus.

Aim 2 – objectives

- After the home visit has been carried out, Mrs X will take an active role in decision-making with regard to the adaptations recommended by the therapist.
- Mrs X will practise bath transfers using a shower board in the occupational therapy department bathroom, and will learn safe transfer techniques.
- Mrs X will practise stair mobility, with supervision of the therapist.
- Mrs X will progress to independent stair mobility, using a stair rail to aid her balance.
- Mrs X will be aware of stair safety.

Aim 3 – objectives

- Mrs X will try out various items of assistive equipment in hospital.
- Mrs X will liaise with the therapist with regard to which items she views meet her needs.

- Mrs X will learn adaptive techniques, where necessary, in order to facilitate independent dressing.

Aim 4 – objectives

- Mrs X will read information provided by the therapist regarding one-handed computer keyboards.
- Mrs X will undertake the responsibility of accessing an adaptive keyboard, should she wish to use one to assist with her work role.

Aim 5 – objectives

- Mrs X will acknowledge and express her concerns regarding the change in her body image.
- Mrs X will acknowledge and express her concerns regarding the changes in her functional capabilities.
- Mrs X will read information provided by the therapist, detailing various support groups for amputees.
- Mrs X will undertake the responsibility of making contact with her chosen support end groups for details of meetings.

SELECTION, ANALYSIS AND APPLICATION OF ACTIVITIES

A large part of the intervention plan for Mrs X was concerned with activities of daily living; this was consistent with her self-identified needs. This encompasses both client-centred and rehabilitative theories. Rehabilitation focuses on enabling individuals to function in ways that are meaningful to them, in line with their capabilities and interests. Enabling clients to participate in everyday activities also facilitates a sense of normality and familiarity (Bye, 1998).

As part of the initial assessment, the therapist asked Mrs X to walk a short distance on the ward, and to perform bed, chair, bath and toilet transfers. Through discussion with Mrs X and through analysis of her mobility and transfers, it was apparent that Mrs X's balance had been altered by the loss of her left arm. With regard to transfers, Mrs X's main problem was with using the bath. She was subsequently seen in the occupational therapy department for further assessment and practise of her transfers, using a shower board. This item of equipment proved successful; the occupational therapist would recommend the provision of a shower board for use at home after discharge to facilitate greater independence and safety when showering.

Due to a reduction in her standing balance, Mrs X practised walking on stairs in the hospital. Through assessment of her stair mobility, it was evident that for Mrs X to walk safely, she needed to use a rail on her right side to provide extra stability. As it had been gathered from the initial assessment that Mrs X's stair rail at home was on the left side ascending, a referral was made to the local social services occupational therapist to recommend installation of a right side rail.

To enable this referral to be made, an access home visit (i.e. without the patient present) was made in order for measurement of Mrs X's stairs. A thorough assessment of Mrs X's home environment was made to highlight any other hazards that may compromise her safety following discharge. However, no other adaptations were deemed necessary. Environmental modification reflects another facet of the rehabilitative frame of reference; it is a compensatory strategy that aims to maximize functional performance (Culler, 1998).

An important aspect of the client-centred approach used was with regard to the provision of resources and information. Mrs X was given a list of compensatory techniques to assist with activities of daily living and also information on companies that manufacture one-handed computer keyboards. Additionally, as she had expressed an interest in joining a support group for amputees, she was provided with a list of relevant organizations. In accordance with the client-centred approach, this placed the client in a position of responsibility (Law *et al.*, 1995); it would be down to Mrs X to contact manufacturers and support groups. In this way, the occupational therapist was simply a facilitator working to enable the client to generate and implement solutions (Law and Mills, 1998). By providing Mrs X with resources and information, the occupational therapist creates an environment that is supportive of change and learning; however, it is the client who actually brings about that change (Pollock and McColl, 1998). One of the intervention sessions involved the occupational therapist giving Mrs X the opportunity to try out various pieces of equipment that are available, to assist with daily living tasks. Mrs X had the opportunity to test a button hook and also elastic shoelaces, which proved to meet her needs in assisting her with problem areas of her self-care. In addition, Mrs X was shown items such as Dycem matting (to provide a non-slip surface for stabilizing objects), a Nelson knife (a combined knife and fork in one, for one-handed eating), plate surrounds, a Spillnot (to enable one-handed opening of jars and bottles) a work station (a chopping board comprising a spike for anchoring vegetables down for ease of one-handed chopping) and a buttering board.

Cooper (1997) suggests that the provision of equipment can have an essential role in the rehabilitative process; occupational therapists should recognize its positive aspects, i.e. that it is enabling, and can encourage clients to gain a sense of control and independence. Through educating clients about the equipment available, they are able to make informed choices and decisions about which ones will best meet their needs (Law *et al.*, 1995).

Mrs X was seen in the occupational therapy department kitchen for a combined assessment and treatment session that involved her making a hot drink.

This intervention was intended to address not only functional capabilities, but also the psychological difficulties commonly experienced by new amputees as they attempt to adapt to their new situation. It had been noted through intervention sessions, and also through liaison with ward staff, that Mrs X appeared low in mood following her surgery. Because making a hot drink was an achievable task for Mrs X, it allowed her to feel effective and competent (Baum, 1998), thus improving her confidence and self-esteem. Also, enabling disabled clients to meet their personal goals can help them to enlarge their scope of values so that physique is less important than what one can do and be (Yerxa, 1996). Mayers (1990) writes that part of the uniqueness of occupational therapy is that it addresses client's psychosocial, emotional and spiritual needs; it is holistic. A key skill in the occupational therapist's repertoire is to recognize that limited mobility does not just affect the client's ability to function in the physical environment, but that it affects all areas of the client's life.

Mrs X had expressed the importance of being able to resume her role of meal provider to her family. This led to two scheduled kitchen sessions, in order to allow Mrs X to work on tasks that were directly relevant to her lifestyle (Culler, 1998) and practise for real-life situations (Jonsson et al., 1999). One of the goals of cancer rehabilitation is to improve the quality of survival in order that clients not only regain independence, but also their productivity (Strong, 1987).

Hot drink preparation provided Mrs X with an opportunity to practise kitchen tasks, for the first time, as an amputee. This intervention provided a protected, safe environment, with all the previously seen assistive equipment around her, as well as the presence of the occupational therapist. It also gave Mrs X the opportunity to be able to express concerns regarding her safety and her competence in the kitchen.

The contraindications of this task were related to fatigue and balance. To address the issue of fatigue, Mrs X was provided with a perching stool to enable her to sit down in between components of the task, thus conserving energy. Energy conservation was an important aspect to consider, as Mrs X's activity tolerance was fairly limited, and also because it can be beneficial in reducing pain (Cooper, 1997). Reduced balance had an effect on Mrs X's safety in the kitchen, particularly when bending down to get the milk from the refrigerator. To address this problem, Mrs X was advised to sit on a perching stool and then bend forward to reach items, rather than bend from a standing position. This technique was tried and proved successful. Additionally, Mrs X was provided with an Easireach to enable her to reach packets from low cupboards, to avoid her having to bend too far. These compensatory devices and techniques increased both Mrs X's safety and independence in the kitchen. Such teaching–learning processes represent an integral part of occupational therapy (Bain, 1998).

As Mrs X was able to prepare a hot drink independently, she was seen on a subsequent occasion in the occupational therapy department kitchen to practise preparing a meal. She chose to cook spaghetti bolognese, a meal that she regularly prepared for her family premorbidly. The ingredients required were purchased on her behalf by the occupational therapist. Mrs X made use of the devices available in the kitchen to enable her to chop an onion independently, to steady items on the worktop, and to open the jar of bolognese sauce. Again, Mrs X used the perching stool, in order to rest between task components, and also the technique previously shown to her to access refrigerated items. In addition, she used a kitchen trolley to transport the finished meal to the table. Again, Mrs X demonstrated independence in carrying out kitchen tasks, with the use of compensatory techniques and devices.

Subsequent to the above interventions, a referral was made to Mrs X's local social services occupational therapist to recommend provision of the following equipment, to facilitate increased independence and safety post-discharge:

- shower board
- stair rail (right side ascending)
- perching stool
- kitchen trolley.

ACTIVITY ANALYSIS

This activity analysis is based on Baum et al.'s model (1998). This model of activity analysis was chosen as it is consistent with the COMP; it addresses the cognitive and physical capabilities of the individual, and acknowledges environmental considerations. It is also holistic in that it considers the psychosocial elements of activity.

ACTIVITY: COOKING SPAGHETTI

ACTIVITY PROCESS

1. Activity of: productivity;
   Appropriateness: activity is appropriate to Mrs X's lifestyle and interests
   Sequence involved:
   Step 1: get saucepan out of cupboard;
   Step 2: fill saucepan with boiling water;
   Step 3: place saucepan on hob;
   Step 4: turn cooker on at mains;
   Step 5: set hob to correct setting;
   Step 6: weigh out spaghetti;
   Step 7: when water boils, put spaghetti into pan;
   Step 8: allow water to return to boil;
   Step 9: allow 10 minutes for spaghetti to cook;

Step 10: turn off hob;

Step 11: drain cooked spaghetti;

Step 12: put cooked spaghetti onto plate.

2. Ingredients required: water, pasta;
3. Tools and equipment required: saucepan, cooker, colander, kitchen scales, kitchen timer;
4. Safety precautions: awareness of dangers associated with using cooker and also of boiling water.

ENVIRONMENTAL CONSIDERATIONS

1. Furniture and positioning: perching stool can be positioned close to cooker, in order that Mrs X can sit down in between components of the task, to assist with energy conservation;
2. External stimulation: good level of lighting required, to ensure safety;
3. Auditory: there should be no distractions.

CHARACTERISTICS OF ACTIVITY

1. Physical:
   - can be performed one-handed;
   - can be performed in a seated position (using a perching stool);
   - requires upper limb strength to transport full saucepan;
   - must be able to pronate wrist in order to be able to drain pasta into colander;
   - requires mainly gross motor control;
   - requires eye–hand coordination;
   - requires weight-bearing ability in lower limbs;
   - requires ability to perform sit-to-stand transfers;
   - requires standing and sitting balance;
   - requires trunk control for sitting;
   - needs to be able to walk short distance to sink while carrying saucepan;
   - requires manual dexterity for opening spaghetti packet.
2. Sensory awareness required:
   - touch: hot;
   - sight: to be able to use scales, and cooker controls;
   - sound: required if using timer;
   - taste: for gratification at end of task.
3. Perceptual skills required:
   - body scheme
   - figure ground
   - kinaesthesia
   - spatial relationships

- motor planning
- proprioception.
4. Cognitive skills required:
   - concentration
   - short-term memory
   - problem solving
   - sequencing
   - safety and judgement
   - basic numeracy to use scales, and timer
   - decision-making skills – in order to select meal to be prepared.
5. Psychosocial factors involved:
   - probability for success
   - confidence building
   - increased sense of self-efficacy
   - gratification at end of task
   - client is in a position of control and decision-making.
6. Social interaction:
   - task to be performed by client, with therapist and OT student present in kitchen;
   - finished meal can be shared with staff.
7. Promotion of goals, motivation and interest:
   - promotes independence
   - gives client a sense of control
   - builds confidence
   - fulfils Mrs X's productivity needs
   - relevant to Mrs X's lifestyle
   - skills can be transferred to the home environment.

POTENTIAL FOR GRADING

The task of meal preparation can be graded to increase demand on the client's physical and cognitive abilities (Young and Quinn, 1992). Demand on the client's functional abilities can be increased through the use of more complex recipes, combining meal preparation with simultaneous hot drink preparation, component tasks that require more fine motor control and grip strength and undertaking a meal that takes longer to prepare (to increase demand for activity tolerance). Meal preparation can be graded to make it a less demanding task through the use of simpler recipes (i.e. with fewer steps to follow, and involving fewer complicated techniques), assistive equipment and verbal prompting.

GRADING AND MODIFICATION

Grading of individual activities was not necessary for Mrs X, as she demonstrated competency in the tasks she was required to perform. However, the kitchen tasks were graded – she began with a simple task (i.e. making a hot drink) and progressed onto the more complex meal preparation task. Modification was implemented through the use of compensatory techniques and assistive devices to increase independence and safety.

EVALUATION OF ACTIVITIES AND INTERVENTION

One way in which the outcomes of the interventions were measured was through client feedback. For example, following both of the kitchen assessments, Mrs X reported to the occupational therapist that carrying out these tasks had greatly improved her confidence in this area. She reported that she felt competent in the kitchen, and also safe, having been shown compensatory techniques and devices. Such experiences of a sense of self-efficacy can aid clients to gain in motivation, which, in turn, contributes to improved occupational performance and well-being (Baum, 1998).

Mrs X was reassessed on the ward following her readmission to hospital, rather than through a home visit, as originally planned. She reported that no new problems had arisen during the time she spent at home and that she found all the equipment useful and did not identify any further needs. She had achieved the level of independence intended in the therapeutic objectives set.

The interventions used are in accordance with the World Health Organization's global strategy for cancer, which emphasizes the importance of the provision of education and information for individuals with cancer. This strategy also stresses the importance of a holistic approach within healthcare, in order that psychosocial issues are recognized as well as medical and functional ones (WHO, 2000). Similarly, the Calman–Hine report has suggested that the psychosocial aspects of cancer should be considered at all stages of healthcare delivery (Calman and Hine, 1995).

Research has shown that elements of the client-centred approach, such as 'respectful and supportive services . . . and information exchange', can generate improved client satisfaction (Law et al., 1995, p. 255). The intervention plan used with Mrs X can be said to have been successful in that it enabled her to obtain a sense of satisfaction from carrying out activities of daily living (Jonsson et al., 1999). Historically, the outcome of cancer services has been measured in terms of survival (Calman and Hine, 1995) but it has been recognized that quality of life is of high importance.

It would have been useful, and appropriate, to have used the Canadian Occupational Performance Measure (COPM) with Mrs X. As an initial assessment tool, the COPM ensures that clients' roles are recognized, and subsequently encompassed in the treatment plan; this tool ensures that interventions are meaningful to the client, through enabling the therapist to gain an understanding of the occupations in which they are typically engaged. Because it is such an individualized tool, the COPM is useful at the re-evaluation stage of the occupational therapy process (Pollock et al., 1999). It can be used to re-evaluate goals (Sumsion, 1999) and it facilitates a flexible and dynamic therapeutic process, as it can highlight changes in performance aspirations and satisfaction (Pollock *et al.*, 1999).

The COPM can be used in the first instance to generate a baseline score of the clients' perception of their performance, and their satisfaction with that performance. Another score can then be recorded at reassessment, to be used as an outcome measure, to evaluate the appropriateness, effectiveness and efficiency of the service delivered (Foto, 1996). As it was, the outcome of intervention with Mrs X was given in a highly narrative, qualitative form.

A key aspect of the occupational therapist's role with this client group is with regard to close liaison with members of the multiprofessional team, which included the physiotherapist, social worker, ward nursing staff, and a specialist nurse from the psychological medicine team. A collaborative approach is essential, in order that clients experience continuity of care (Cooper, 1997). This also concurs with the government's plan to increase the standards of care for cancer patients, by encouraging the streamlining of various services (Department of Health, 2000), and the Calman–Hine report, which also stresses the importance of multidisciplinary team working (Calman and Hine, 1995).

SUMMARY AND RECOMMENDATIONS

Mrs X is a 55-year-old woman, recently discharged home from hospital, following a left forequarter amputation, performed with the intention of curing her from a soft tissue sarcoma of the left axilla. Unfortunately, Mrs X was readmitted 10 days after this discharge, as she began to experience generalized chest pains. On readmission to hospital, a CT (computed tomography) scan showed the presence of metastases in the upper left lobe of the lungs and also the liver. Currently, Mrs X is living independently at home, pending the commencement of further chemotherapy.

The hospital occupational therapist is not currently involved in Mrs X's case, but is likely to become involved again if she is readmitted, to reassess her functional abilities. Mrs X is currently on a waiting list at another specialist hospital for provision of a left upper limb prosthesis. Ongoing emotional support will be available to Mrs X, provided by the hospital's psychological medicine team, on an outpatient basis. Her children will also continue to receive emotional support and counselling to help them to adapt to their mother's disability and recurrent disease.

REFERENCES

Bain, B. (1998) Treatment of Performance Contexts. *Occupational Therapy*, 9th edn (eds M. E. Neistadt and E. B. Crepeau), Lippincott, Philadelphia, PA.

Barraclough, J. (1994) *Cancer and Emotion: A Practical Guide to Psycho-oncology*, 2nd edn, Wiley and Sons, Chichester.

Baum, C. (1998) Client-centred Practice in a Changing Health Care System. *Client-Centred Occupational Therapy* (ed. M. Law), Slack, New Jersey.

Baum, C. M., Bass-Haugen, J. and Christiansen, C. (1998) Person-Environment-Occupation-Performance: A Model for Planning Interventions for Individuals and Organizations. *Client-centred Occupational Therapy* (ed. M. Law), Slack, New Jersey.

Burt, C. M. and Smith, P. (1996) Work Evaluation and Work Hardening. *Occupational Therapy: Practice Skills for Physical Dysfunction*, 4th edn (ed. L. W. Pedretti), Mosby, St Louis.

Bye, R. A. (1998) When clients are dying: Occupational therapists' perspectives. *Occupational Therapy Journal of Research*, **18**(1), 3–24.

Calman, K. and Hine, D. (1995) *A Policy Framework for Commissioning Cancer Services*, Department of Health, London.

Cancerlink (2001) *Talking to Children when an Adult has Cancer*, 4th edn, Cancerlink, London.

Colburn, J. and Ibbotson, V. (1992) Upper Limb Amputees and Limb Deficient Children. *Occupational Therapy and Physical Dysfunction: Principles, Skills and Practice* (eds A. Turner, M. Foster and S. E. Johnson), Churchill Livingstone, Edinburgh.

Cooper, J. (1997) *Occupational Therapy in Oncology and Palliative Care*, Whurr, London.

Culler, K. H. (1998) Treatment of Work and Productive Activities, Home and Family Management. *Occupational Therapy*, 8th edn (eds H. L. Hopkins and H. D. Smith), Lippincott, Philadelphia, PA.

Culler, K. H. (1998) *Willard and Spackman's Occupational Therapy*, 9th edn (eds M. E. Neistadt and E. B. Crepeau), Lippincott, Philadelphia, PA.

Department of Health (2000) *NHS Cancer Plan*: www.doh.gov.uk/cancer

Dutton, R. (1995) *Clinical Reasoning in Physical Disabilities*, Williams and Wilkins, Baltimore, MD.

Faulkner, A. and Maguire, P. (1994) *Talking to Cancer Patients and Their Families*, Oxford University Press, Oxford.

Fisher, K. and Hanspal, R. S. (1998) Phantom pain, anxiety, depression, and their relation in consecutive patients with amputated limbs: Case reports. *British Medical Journal*, **316**(7135), 903–4.

Foster, M. (1992) Theoretical Frameworks. *Occupational Therapy and Physical Dysfunction: Principles, Skills and Practice*, 3rd edn (eds A. Turner, M. Foster and S. E. Johnson), Churchill Livingstone, Edinburgh.

Foto, M. (1996) Outcome studies: The what, why, how and when. *American Journal of Occupational Therapy*, **50**(2), 87–8.

Goffman, E. (1968) *Stigma: Notes on the Management of Spoiled Identity*, Penguin, Harmondsworth.

Greaves, M. (2000) *Cancer: The Evolutionary Legacy*, Oxford University Press, Oxford.

Guex, P. (1994) *An Introduction to Psycho-oncology*, Routledge, London.

Hammell, K. W. (1998) Client-centred occupational therapy: Collaborative planning, accountable intervention. *Client-Centred Occupational Therapy* (ed. M. Law), Slack, New Jersey.

Jonsson, A. L. T., Moller, A. and Grimby, G. (1999) Managing occupations in every-day life to achieve adaptation. *American Journal of Occupational Therapy*, **53**(7), 353–62.

Law, M., Baptiste, S., Carswell, A., McColl, M. A., Polatajko, H. and Pollock, N. (1994) *Canadian Occupational Performance Measure*, Canadian Association of Occupational Therapy Publications, Toronto.

Law, M., Baptiste, S. and Mills, J. (1995) Client-centred practice: What does it mean and does it make a difference? *Canadian Journal of Occupational Therapy*, **62**(5), 250–7.

Law, M. and Mills, J. (1998) *Client-Centred Occupational Therapy* (ed. M. Law), Slack, New Jersey.

Law, M., Polatajko, H., Baptiste, S. and Townsend, E. (1997). *Enabling Occupation: An Occupational Therapy Perspective* (ed. E. Towsend), CAOT Publications, Ottawa.

Lloyd, C. and Coggles, L. (1990) Psychosocial issues for people with cancer and their families. *Canadian Journal of Occupational Therapy*, **57**(4), 211–15.

Maguire, P. and Parkes, C. M. (1998) Coping with loss: Surgery and loss of body parts. *British Medical Journal*, **316**(7137), 1068–88.

Mayers, C. A. (1990) A philosophy unique to occupational therapy. *British Journal of Occupational Therapy*, **53**(9), 379–80.

McColl, M. A., Gerein, N. and Valentine, F. (1997) *Occupational Therapy: Enabling function and well being*, 2nd edn (eds C. Christiansen and C. Baum), Slack, New Jersey.

McColl, M. A., Gerein, N. and Valentine, F. (2005) Occupational Therapy Interventions in a Rehabilitation context. *Occupational Therapy: Performance, Participation & Well-Being*, 3rd edn (eds Christiansen, C. H., Baum. C. and Bass-Haugen, J.), Slack: New Jersey.

Mock, V. (1993) Body image in women treated for breast cancer. *Nursing Research*, **42**(3), 153–7.

Neistadt, M. E. (2000) *Occupational Therapy Evaluation for Adults: A pocket guide*, Lippincott, Williams and Wilkins, Baltimore, MD.

Newell, R. (2000) *Body Image and Disfigurement Care*, Routledge, London.

Parkes, C. M. (1998) Coping with loss: The dying adult. *British Medical Journal*, **316**(7140), 1313–15.

Pollock, N. and McColl, M. A. (1998) Assessment in Client-centred Occupational Therapy. *Client-Centred Occupational Therapy* (ed. M. Law), Slack, New Jersey.

Price, M. (2000) *Phantom Pain*: accessed at www.limblessassociation.co.uk

Sarafino, E. P. (1998) *Health Psychology: Biopsychosocial interactions*, 3rd edn, John Wiley and Sons, New York.

Scambler, G. (1997) *Sociology as Applied to Medicine*, W.B. Saunders, Edinburgh.

Seidel, A. C. (1998) Theories Derived from Rehabilitation Perspectives. *Occupational Therapy*, 9th edn (eds M. E. Neistadt and E. B. Crepeau), Lippincott, Philadelphia, PA.

Souhami, R. and Tobias, J. (1995) *Cancer and its Management*, 2nd edn, Blackwell Science, Oxford.

Strong, J. (1987) Occupational therapy and cancer rehabilitation. *British Journal of Occupational Therapy*, **50**(1), 4–6.

Sumsion, T. (ed.) (1999) *Client-Centred Occupational Therapy: A guide to implementation*. Churchill Livingstone, Edinburgh.

Taylor, S. E. (1995) *Health Psychology*, 3rd edn, McGraw-Hill, New York.

Vachon, M. L. S. (1998) Emotional problems in palliative care: patient, family and professional. *Oxford Textbook of Palliative Medicine* (eds D. Doyle, G. W. C. Hanks and N. Macdonald), Oxford University Press, Oxford.

World Health Organization (2000) *Developing a Global Strategy for Cancer*: www.who.int/ncd/cancer/strategy

Yerxa, E. J. (1996) The Social and Psychological Experience of Having a Disability. *Occupational Therapy: Practice skills for physical dysfunction*, 4th edn (ed. L. W. Pedretti), Mosby, St Louis, MO.

Young, M. E. and Quinn, E. (1992) *Theories and Principles of Occupational Therapy*, Churchill Livingstone, Edinburgh.

Zabalegui, A. (1999) Coping strategies and psychological distress in patients with advanced cancer. *Oncology Nursing Forum*, **26**(9), 1511–18.

8 Occupational Therapy in Paediatric Oncology and Palliative Care

CLAIRE TESTER

Children are not meant to die, they are our hope. They are to live on into the future and, after a full life to die at an old age. It goes against our understanding of the world order if a child dies. When a child is diagnosed with a life-limiting condition, the world falls in on the parents and family and, although adults may think the child is unaware, the world falls in on the child too. The normality of family life is shattered and the emotional strain, anxiety and fear of when death will occur is held within the family, often silently.

In this chapter the impact upon the child and family will be considered, and the role of the occupational therapist will be discussed. Although it is often thought that cancer is the main life-limiting condition affecting children, this is not the case: there are other life-limiting conditions which are discussed later in this chapter. The term 'child' will be used throughout but this does not exclude infants or adolescents.

PAEDIATRIC PALLIATIVE CARE

It is unsettling for the term palliative care to be applied to children when it is understood that there is no cure (Mosby, 1999) and the child will die. When children are referred for palliative care it does not mean that they are in their terminal phase and that death is imminent. Palliative care is working with the child and family to support them in every way possible emotionally, practically and psychologically in making the most of the time they have together and to help them come to terms with what is happening at each stage of the condition, including the terminal stage, at death and in bereavement. The focus is on the child and family and their needs, which are constantly changing. The approach differs from the usual therapeutic approach of working towards improvement, independence and discharge because the child deteriorates, losing skills over time, and is not discharged. The palliative paediatric

Occupational Therapy in Oncology and Palliative Care. Edited by J. Cooper
© 2006 John Wiley & Sons Ltd

occupational therapist adopts a broad view to include the child and family, utilizing a wide range of skills and expertise, and focuses on the quality of life including symptom control, with an open and sensitive approach (Addington-Hall and Higginson, 2001).

> Palliative care is the active total care of the child's body, mind and spirit, and also involves giving support to the family. Health providers must evaluate and alleviate a child's physical, psychological, and social distress. Effective palliative care requires a broad multi-disciplinary approach that includes the family and makes use of available community resources; it can be provided in tertiary care facilities, in community health centres and even in children's homes.
>
> (WHO, 1990)

Depending upon the diagnosis and prognosis, children of all ages may be referred for palliative care. The timing of this is dependent upon the health of the child, the needs of the family for support and the stage of the condition. The course of the condition may vary from a few days, to months or several years. For example, the prognosis for babies with infantile Battens disease can be a few months and palliative care therefore begins immediately.

Specialist palliative care may be provided by a children's hospice, or a combination of existing therapy and service provision with hospice stays and returns to hospital and/or home. Each child is unique and never more so than in palliative care. Although the field of paediatric palliative care is relatively new, occupational therapists have long worked with children with life-limiting conditions in the community and clinics as part of an active caseload. This is still the case as the majority of children with life-limiting conditions live at home and attend nursery or school and are involved in therapy programmes with the support of the occupational therapist. Normality is maintained as far as possible for the child and family, encompassing activities of daily living, mobility, accessing the school curriculum, being able to play, whether early play or participating in sport, and social and leisure activities. A community paediatric occupational therapist and a social services occupational therapist may be working with a child and their family for some time before the child is referred to a hospice with a paediatric palliative occupational therapist. This means that the community occupational therapist needs to adopt a palliative care approach.

WHEN PALLIATIVE CARE BEGINS

There is no distinct point at which a child or teenager requires palliative care as opposed to curative care (see Figure 8.1). A child with a life-limiting condition is not necessarily directly referred for palliative care. The emphasis is

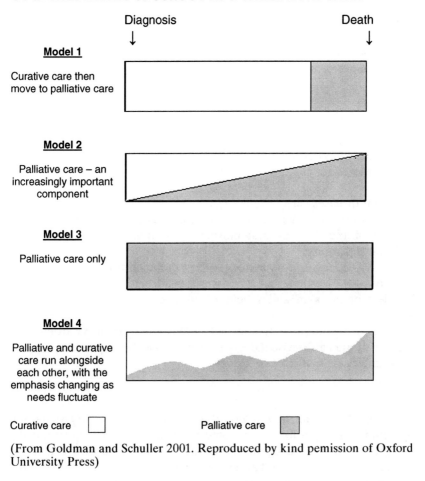

Diagnosis   Death

Model 1

Curative care then
move to palliative care

Model 2

Palliative care – an
increasingly important
component

Model 3

Palliative care only

Model 4

Palliative and curative
care run alongside
each other, with the
emphasis changing as
needs fluctuate

Curative care   ☐   Palliative care   ▨

(From Goldman and Schuller 2001. Reproduced by kind pemission of Oxford
University Press)

Figure 8.1 Model of curative and palliative care relationships

upon support and the needs of the child and the family. This changes and this
is the main factor in referral for palliative care. However, being referred for
palliative care does not exclude other therapies that can continue.

Palliative care can be seen to carry on alongside active therapy. It is as the
child's condition deteriorates that palliative care increases. The time frame
differs for each child depending on the course of his or her condition. For
some children their deterioration is gradual, becoming sensory-impaired and
losing motor skills as in Nieman Pick syndrome. With cancer there can be a
sudden deterioration over a short time, or a gradual deterioration over a
longer time depending on the growth of the tumour and its response to treatment. Depending upon the child's condition and its progression, palliative

care may extend from the point of diagnosis, e.g. Battens disease, or may be when curative treatment has failed, e.g. cancer. Children with complex and combined conditions may be referred for palliative care when their health deteriorates and is compromised, e.g. severe cerebral palsy with intractable epilepsy.

CONDITIONS

Cancer is often considered to be the main life-limiting condition affecting children but there are:

- malignant diseases such as leukodystrophy;
- metabolic disorders such as mucopolysaccharides, e.g. Sanfilippo;
- diseases of the nervous system such as Battens disease, Duchenne muscular dystrophy;
- diseases of the respiratory system such as cystic fibrosis;
- chromosomal disorders such as Edwards syndrome (trisomy 18)
- disorders of the skin and subcutaneous tissues such as epidermolysis bullosa;
- disorders of the immune system such as Wiscott Aldrich syndrome;
- diseases of the cardiovascular system such as cardiac myopathy;
- organ failure such as liver or kidney.

(Goldman and Schuller, 2001)

The conditions listed can be diagnosed at birth or in the early years and developmental delay is a feature of some of these conditions. Occasionally children present with rare conditions which cannot be diagnosed easily. Cancer can occur at any age and affect seemingly healthy children and young adults. Treatment for cancer begins immediately and is delivered through the oncology clinics, wards and by the oncology team who make home visits. The cancer may be eradicated or 'cured' but not always. Therefore parents and some teenagers will talk of 'luck' or 'bad luck' in relation to success in treatment. Children do not encounter children with other life-limiting conditions except when admitted to a children's hospice, which is in itself an admission that the child is dying and the treatment has not been successful.

IMPACT ON THE PARENTS AT REFERRAL OF A LIFE-LIMITED CHILD

In order to plan a sensitive approach, it is important for the occupational therapist to consider the child and family in some depth. There are many psychosocial factors that need to be taken into account including cultural and religious beliefs and how they perceive their child's condition. The time of diagnosis is usually the time the prognosis is also given. This may be just after the baby's birth, months or even years later in the child's life, as in cancer. The age of the child when the prognosis is given is crucial to the understanding of the parent–child attachment relationship, and of the child's emotional and intellectual understanding of what is happening around him or her. Whether there are siblings in the family, and the ages of any siblings, also impacts for they contribute to the family dynamic.

If the prognosis is given around the time of the birth the parents are thrown into the loss of and grieving for the healthy baby they had hoped for. They have to come to terms with this and to bond with the baby they have, and to further adjust to the baby dying. As one mother said, 'I feel so guilty bringing my baby into the world to die so soon.' The loss and grief begin at the time of diagnosis. Anticipatory grief is the mourning behaviour which begins before the child dies (Cook *et al.*, 1973).

> It's like standing on sand, nothing is certain anymore except that my child will die, and I think about it all of the time, knowing that all of the days are going and I can do nothing about it. I cry at night so that she cannot see but it is so painful. I know she's going to go. (A mother of a 7-year-old with leukodystrophy)

Sometimes a prognosis is given and the child surprises everyone by living on. As one 13-year-old boy said two years after being given a prognosis of two months, 'I know doctors can get it wrong. They didn't know that I wasn't ready to die.' Often there is a sense of guilt held by one or both parents. In Duchenne muscular dystrophy the mother is the carrier; this can lead to blame upon the mother by the father and anger from the son. The emotional, physical and often financial strain upon the marital relationship cannot be underestimated. Any difficulty or fragility in the relationship is exacerbated (Grinyer, 2002) and can lead to break-up which in turn causes further distress. The inevitable rounds of clinical visits and tests make their demands upon the entire family as well as the individuals involved. There is pressure of time; of getting to the hospital or specialist clinic (not usually local) while other children in the family need collecting from school or to be dropped off at after school activities. Parents have to take time off from work, which may incur a financial loss. Into this mix staff in the community are introduced. This includes the occupational therapist. The occupational therapist needs to plan visits to suit the child and family. As one mother admitted, 'We hid behind the sofa when the occupational therapist came as we'd already seen the nurse and the physiotherapist that day and we just wanted a break.' A key worker system is helpful for the family in identifying needs and to help colleagues coordinate visits to the family. Communication amongst the multiprofessional team is crucial.

IMPACT ON THE REFERRED CHILD

It is painful but necessary to consider the emotional experience of the referred child or young adult in the midst of all this. The child undergoes tests, injections, swallows the medicine, encounters different professionals, stays in strange environments such as hospital or hospice, loses skills, has a change in routine and becomes the focus of attention for parents and family. As one teenager put it, 'Suddenly everyone is so nice all of the time. It's not normal.'

Children and young adults are sensitive to the fact that their parents are distressed and can see themselves as a cause of further upset for the parent. They enter into an emotional double bind in that they smile and appear content as if unaware of any imminent threat to their life when they are with the parent but feel increasingly isolated and alone with their morbid thoughts and anxieties and present differently when away from a parent. 'John (14) and I never discussed the fact that he was dying, because he knew and I knew and he knew that I knew what was happening. He did not want to hurt us and he did not want to discuss what was happening, and that was alright' (mother's account, Kubler-Ross, 1985).

The normal daily routine can be lost and anxiety heightened. Children and young adults can regress emotionally to an earlier needy stage, and there may be changes in behaviour, e.g. frustration and anger. Consequently such children may be described as difficult. Lansdown (1987) identified five stages a dying child with cancer experiences:

- I am very sick;
- I have an illness that can kill people;
- I have an illness that can kill children;
- I may not get better;
- I am dying.

Bereavement is only considered after death but for the child or young adult who experiences the realization that the treatment is not working and that there is no cure, there is a real sense of loss of their own life while they are alive, and they grieve. This follows the pattern of denial, anger, bargaining, depression, acceptance (Kubler-Ross, 1969) and readjustment. Grieving can also be experienced for each skill lost, e.g. as in Duchenne muscular dystrophy when a teenage boy becomes increasingly dependent as he becomes paralysed while his peers become increasingly independent and active. Children have different concepts of death depending upon their age and this affects their understanding of what is happening to them. The teenager can feel isolated whereas the child aged between two and five does not see death as being permanent (Johnson-Stroderberg, 1981). Understandably, parents find it unbearable to have to consider their child's death or to answer their child's questions. It is necessary for the therapist to ask what children understand about their condition before answering questions or discussing future equipment needs. It is helpful to ascertain what the parents wish their child to know, and perhaps the terms they have used. The family's religious belief may also determine this.

For some children, including infants, their developmental delay means that it is uncertain how much they know about their prognosis. However, they are very aware of how they are feeling and can become anxious and uncomfortable. Anxious parents can increase their sense of insecurity. Children who cannot initiate movement and may have sensory impairment benefit greatly from a sensitive approach and therapy.

IMPACT ON THE SIBLINGS

The focus in the family changes from trying to meet everyone's needs equally to having to attend to one member of the family. Siblings compete for a parent's attention and can feel left out and secondary. The siblings can interpret this as being 'less loved' (Kew, 1975). The age of the siblings determines their level of understanding of the situation and their emotional reaction to it. When introducing play ideas for the referred child it is helpful to include younger siblings as well.

Aspects of normality are important to siblings, especially for teenagers. Having a concrete ramp to the front door and a disabled parking bay outside the house are distinctly 'uncool'. This can cause friction and resentment within the household. Such things cannot be avoided but do need to be explained. Some teenage siblings may distance themselves from the disability associated with the family, and may not bring friends back home. In contrast, some siblings become secondary carers and help parents in this role within the home. This, too, can be difficult as the siblings' own needs can be overlooked within the family.

As palliative care encompasses the whole family, these are some considerations for the occupational therapist. This contributes to an informed and compassionate approach with the emphasis on initially developing trust and helps to determine the starting point for the occupational therapist with the family.

THE ROLE OF THE OCCUPATIONAL THERAPIST

WHICH OCCUPATIONAL THERAPIST?

Referral to an occupational therapist can be confusing for a family; the referred child may see an occupational therapist on the ward of a hospital where the child or teenager is having a prolonged stay, while still maintaining an occupational therapist in the community at school or at home. In addition, an occupational therapist from social services is often involved for specific equipment and/or adaptations for the home. Some oncology teams have their own occupational therapist who will be working with a child and family, and there may be an occupational therapist at the children's hospice. The degree of involvement by the community occupational therapist lessens as the child deteriorates and the paediatric palliative care occupational therapist becomes more involved. There is no definitive point at which the community occupational therapist hands over to the palliative care occupational therapist. The emphasis changes depending on the needs of the child and family, and the course of the condition (see Figure 8.1, p. 109). Both liaise with the social services occupational therapist.

ASSESSMENT

In the normal course of paediatric occupational therapy standardized assessments are carried out and scored, identifying the need for occupational therapy intervention and setting objectives with the child and parent as realistic goals to achieve. There is ongoing review and a reassessment to identify improvement and goals obtained. The child is then discharged.

In paediatric palliative care the approach is different because the child will not improve and is not discharged. In oncology there may be improvement. The occupational therapist has a unique contribution to make through the holistic approach of viewing both the physical impact and the psychological and emotional impact of a condition upon the child and family.

It must be remembered that the child will have undergone many different tests and scans in order for a diagnosis and prognosis to have been reached before encountering the occupational therapist who needs to conduct an assessment. Assessments are used to provide a sound baseline from which the therapist can work by determining the child's skills and identifying needs. However, some may be counterproductive, and the occupational therapist must consider how helpful the assessments may be, not just to herself, but to the child and family. When working with a child with a life-limiting condition, a formal assessment is not always helpful or valid. It is not in the child's interests to have skills measured and scored with a standardized assessment because, when the child or teenager is losing skills, a formal assessment can only highlight this fact. Such an assessment sets up failure as the score will always be down. The occupational therapist must think carefully about what they are trying to assess and how to go about it. There are different models which may be used:

- Developmental – helpful for infants and young children, and children who have profound developmental delay;

- MOHO (Model of Human Occupation) (Kielhofner, 2002) – to help identify what is meaningful. This model needs to be modified with children. Care must be taken in planning unrealistic goals;
- Psychodynamic – looking at the emotional and psychological factors and using these as a basis for approach;
- Biomechanical – when the focus is on activities of daily living and functional activity.

These approaches are often used in conjunction with each other.

In the initial stages sensory integration assessments, such as the Movement Assessment Battery for Children (Movement ABC) may be helpful as a contribution to diagnosis (Henderson *et al.*, 1992). Also the Goodenough-Harris Drawing Test (Goodenough and Harris, 1963), Frostig Developmental Test of Visual Perception (Frostig *et al.*, 1963) and other visual perception tests can be helpful in determining neurological function but are not to be continued as the child deteriorates. The Bayley Scales of Infant Development (Bayley, 1993), and the Sheridan Children's Developmental Progress (0–5 yrs) (Sheridan, 2005) are useful for infants and young children. It is the skilled and experienced paediatric occupational therapist who assesses informally but thoroughly. The key is detailed observation of the child through activity, observing both skills and dysfunction. The occupational therapist observes intently while engaging the child actively. It is important to gain a child's trust. For young children it is necessary to gain the trust of the parent first in front of the child before talking and working with the child directly. The occupational therapist needs to be sensitive to this. The occupational therapist can engage a child in play or an activity as part of an informal assessment. It is helpful for the therapist to observe the child at nursery or school setting, interacting in the playground, in the classroom setting and looking at schoolwork.

CASE STUDY

A 10-year-old boy with an astrocytoma (brain tumour) was trying to maintain normality by attending school but when observed closely he did not have the energy to play in the playground with his friends and was trying to conserve his energy. His friends teased him that he was becoming a 'wimp' and he was becoming socially isolated. His school work was affected by the headaches that he would not tell his teacher about. His handwriting deteriorated and as a result he was given extra handwriting practice at break time.

In cancer, the child may experience periods of fatigue and loss of physical skills affecting independence after treatment though this is not necessarily permanent. There are variable levels of ability performance seen in children and young adults with different conditions that can be affected by medication too, nausea and vomiting being common with cancer treatment.

The occupational therapist is always aware of the development and physical growth of the child while there is a simultaneous deterioration. This often involves sensory impairment. As the occupational therapist is working with children who are deteriorating and losing skills, it is necessary to reset aims and to identify what is meaningful to the child or young adult and to the family. This changes throughout the children's lives due to the different stage of the condition, their level of understanding of what is happening to them, and their emotional and developmental stage.

CASE STUDY

Anne is 7 years old and has Sanfilippo, a life-limiting condition presenting with hydrocephalus, developmental delay, difficulties in motor skills and an affected growth pattern. When she was 3 she was very active, running everywhere, without any sense of danger or boundaries, though she had a limited vocabulary. She became slower in her activity and could no longer bear her weight at 5 years. She slowly stopped speaking but could make some sounds when hungry or in discomfort. Her cognitive abilities deteriorated and she wanted only familiar people around her and the same video to watch. She showed little direct engagement with anyone and her sight began to fail.

The occupational therapist assesses using detailed and careful observations, and a sensitive approach. As a child may change from month to month, or even more frequently, then it is necessary to use one's observations at each encounter. The assessment must also include the child's medical and developmental history (Case-Smith, 1998). Occupational therapy intervention may comprise initially the elements listed in Tables 8.1 and 8.2.

Table 8.1 Occupational therapy intervention in paediatric oncology and palliative care

- Response of infant, child or adolescent to you – with interest? disinterest? awareness? eye contact?
- Observation of interaction and responses with main caregiver, usually mother, and responses to others, e.g. staff.
- Physical appearance – tired? drawn? naso-gastric tube? any dressings?
- Muscle tone.
- Communication skills and behaviour, e.g. eye contact, mood, interest, fatigue.
- Positioning – sitting position? able to reposition or support self?
- Range of movement – active, passive. Are there any contractures?
- Equipment being used – wheelchair, bedpan, hoist in evidence?

Table 8.2 Specific areas for occupational therapy assessment in paediatric oncology and palliative care

---

- Developmental stages – A child may be nine years old chronologically but presenting developmentally at 3 months
- Sensorimotor
- Neuromuscular
- Reflex integration
- Sensory awareness
- Coordination
- Strength and endurance
- Sensory integration – core skills: tactile, vestibular, and proprioceptive
- Cognition
- Orientation
- Comprehension
- Physical assessment re range of movement both active and passive
- Emotional well-being? anxious? shy? clingy to parent? detached?
- Pain – total pain (Saunders, 1993) including physical, emotional, psychosocial, spiritual (see p. 118)
- Play/leisure
- Self-help skills
- Equipment including wheelchair, hoist, slings and other equipment to aid independence
- Social activities
- Technological assist e.g. environmental control
- Nursery/school/college/university
- Housing
- Family situation
- What is meaningful to the child

(Bray & Cooper, 2004)

If children or adolescents are able to communicate then the assessment must include their own subjective assessment of their condition (Muhlenhaupt *et al.*, 1999). For the infant a history and further information can be provided by the parent and members of the multidisciplinary team. The occupational therapist needs to think creatively and to problem solve with compassion. This involves thinking with the head and the heart using emotional intelligence (Lewin and Reed, 1998).

Physical pain is often a symptom of a condition and is always associated with cancer. Although the pain will be treated pharmacologically there is an active role for the occupational therapist in alleviating pain. This can often be the initial prompt for occupational therapist involvement. A pain assessment such as the Faces Scale (Wong and Baker, 1988) or the Eland Color Tool (Eland, 1981) may be used with children to help identify physical pain. However, often pain cannot be communicated except through crying and distressed facial expressions or avoidance of touch.

It is through careful assessment of the range of movement, observation of positioning and activity, and establishment of a normal behaviour pattern with parents that pain can be identified. Pain can be alleviated through supportive positioning using a pressure cushion for seating, or positioning to counteract involuntary motor patterns, e.g. supporting children in a flexor position when they have a strong extensor pattern. A functional seating position is not always necessary and can contribute to pain. The choice of buggy, bed mattress and seating can make a difference. Depending upon the age of the child, activity can act as a distraction. Guided imagery and relaxation techniques can be helpful. Parents can be shown how to calm their child or baby actively through touch. Soothing music can be helpful. It is important that the pain is understood and accepted as real and that there is no heroism attached to refusing pain relief. A 12-year-old boy with a spinal tumour on experiencing pain on being moved said, 'I'm sorry Dad. I'm a failure. I will need to take my fentanyl after all. I'm not brave enough.'

Pain should be viewed as 'total' (Saunders, 1993), that is emotional, physical, psychosocial and spiritual. Emotional and spiritual pain are felt acutely but not as obviously. They can be perceived as demanding or difficult behaviour, depression or a heightened state of anxiety. Conversely the teenager may appear keen to please and comply with all requests in order to be the good patient so that all will be made better and normality restored. It is necessary to consider what acts as comfort to the child/teenager and their own need for an emotional container (Bion, 1984). The main caregiver is usually the mother, who acts as a secure base (Bowlby, 1988).

THE MAIN AIMS OF OCCUPATIONAL THERAPY IN PALLIATIVE CARE

- To build on existing skills, and where possible to maintain skills. This may be using aids and equipment, or by finding a different technique to maintain a skill such as playing computer games, or self-feeding.
- To enable the child to achieve. It is important to find out what is meaningful to the child or adolescent. It may not be the practical aspects, e.g. of bathing or dressing, as perceived by parents, but being able to text message on the mobile, or having a sleepover at granny's house with siblings.
- To support by identifying psychosocial and physical needs, and the developmental stage including emotional needs. This includes listening actively to the anxieties of the child or teenager, to encourage self-esteem, possibly to work on social skills, e.g. when there is hair loss, loss of friends, or confinement to a wheelchair. Support is also given to the parents. It is a complex dynamic when strong emotions are unconsciously passed from parent to child and back again. This includes tension and fear. By listening to and tolerating the parent's chaos, it is possible to think about the mental pain without becoming overwhelmed. In this way the parent can be helped to consider their child's own feelings (Fraiberg, 1980).

- To maintain independence. When motor skills are being lost it is essential that teenagers particularly have a sense of independence and control over their own lives. This can include adapted switches for a light, or door, an environmental control system and operating the electric hoist control. They must also make choices and exercise some control over daily activities such as choosing clothes or making their own will.

- To facilitate communication. This ranges from working with parents and their baby to help them recognize the baby's different needs, to calming massage techniques for a parent to give to their child who has neither speech nor movement, to anger management techniques between a parent and teenager to facilitate their talking to each other in a positive way. Therapeutic play and expression through play is helpful for a child who is struggling with anxiety or pain, whether physical or emotional, and is suffering (Brown, 2001). It is not always possible for children or teenagers to have open and supportive dialogue with the parents who are also struggling to come to terms with what is happening to them. As children or teenagers deteriorate and reach their terminal stage, it is important that there is a positive connection between them and their loved ones.

The occupational therapist has a role in assisting referred children to be all that they can be. The way in which the therapy is delivered requires tact. One mother said, 'They ask you what the problem is, you tell them what you are doing, and they say, "Do this. Try that", as if living with someone who is dying can be fixed in some way. It is a total draining experience and has no real end.'

Working with this client group necessitates sensitivity and it is essential that intervention is at the pace and request of the family. The occupational therapist needs to identify the difficulties and the needs of the child, the parent and family. These are often different.

In palliative care the focus is not on the disease and its progression but on the child, the family and their perceptions of the condition and the needs arising (Muhlenhaupt et al., 1999). In children's hospices the occupational therapist is a member of the care team and duties may be extended to changing nappy pads, preparing a room, assisting in active washing and dressing, as well as care of a body after death, moving and handling training, risk assessments and equipment issues within the hospice itself.

COPING MECHANISMS

Different families have different ways of coping. The way in which they do this can affect the occupational therapist. The news of the diagnosis and prognosis can be received as the initial stage of grief, that is shock and denial, leading to anger. These strong emotions can be experienced for a prolonged time. For example, the parents may be in denial refusing therapy input and especially equipment. Equipment in the home can be viewed as a visual and tangible aspect of disability, which is resented. In contrast some parents and teenagers can be perceived as 'demanding', requiring a lot of equipment and input, and focusing on details of what is not right, and perceiving that services and provision are not fair. This is an aspect based in reality when some services find it difficult to make a financial undertaking such as an extension for the home when the child is referred for palliative care. Parents remark that they seem to have 'to fight for everything their child needs'. The fighting and anger may be a way in which some parents feel in control, that they are actively 'doing something positive' when faced with their child's situation in which they feel powerless. This can make it difficult for the occupational therapist, especially the social services occupational therapist, who is assessing and providing equipment for the home and involved in adaptations.

WHEN A CHILD IS DYING

The terminal stage and the length of time at this stage is different for everyone. Sometimes it can be predicted, e.g. in Sanfilippo, but for others it can be brief, e.g. in Duchenne muscular dystrophy, when death may occur through sudden cardiac failure. This also means that the child may be at home, hospital or hospice. Some parents prefer their son or daughter to die at home and to leave the hospital or hospice; for some teenagers the choice has been to die at the hospice. The occupational therapist may be involved in maintaining positional comfort and practical aspects in advice or equipment provision for bathing, etc. Depending upon the role and relationship of the occupational therapist with the child, it may be the occupational therapist to whom they put questions and concerns that they cannot discuss with their parents, such as funeral requests, what will happen at death, and their fears. Such questions occur spontaneously and cannot be anticipated.

The occupational therapist at the hospice may be actively involved in the care of the child at death and immediately afterwards depending upon the relationship with the child and family. This can be a positive experience, helping the parents to bathe and dress their child for the last time, and to talk about their child. At a children's hospice a dead body can be maintained for a few days in a special room set aside with coolers rather than radiators. In this way the family can visit their son or daughter and begin to say goodbye and come to terms with the death.

The hospice occupational therapist may be involved in bereavement support for the family and siblings, which can continue for as long as the family needs it. This varies from several months to several years during which time the family are supported in adjusting to life without their son or daughter. The way in which the child or young adult and family were supported through life can impact the grief process either positively or negatively. Bereaved siblings may experience guilt for feelings they had of resentment while their brother or sister was alive and also hold hidden fears that they will die. 'Every so often he is under the weather, often admits to "bumps and lumps" of unidentified origin and is worried' (mother of bereaved sibling, Grinyer, 2002)

WELL-BEING OF THE THERAPIST

Working with children and teenagers who have a life-limiting condition is challenging work both professionally and personally. The palliative care approach is different from a rehabilitative one as the patients are deteriorating and will die. In paediatric palliative care the children will not reach adulthood, and this is a painful realization for the occupational therapist. There is a lot of pain, both physical and emotional, experienced by the referred child and family resulting in strong feelings that families understandably have difficulty bearing and tolerating. This results in emotions being projected onto those who work with the child and family. Such strong projections can be introjected (Klein, 1998) by the occupational therapist and owned by them, e.g. feelings of inadequacy, of hopelessness, of overwhelming sadness and grief, which can lead to the occupational therapist feeling deskilled. Gammage *et al.* (1976) and Kubler-Ross (1969) conclude that to work in palliative care the occupational therapist needs to have confronted the inevitability of one's own death first.

Parents and children usually talk to someone they feel they can trust and who they see often. This can be the occupational therapist in the community or at the hospice. It is important that the occupational therapist does not transfer his or her own feelings and experiences onto the client but maintains a professional and compassionate approach. A parent whose child is dying is overwhelmed and feels inadequate. If the occupational therapist identifies with the parent, supervision may be necessary, and may come from a psychologist, play therapist or psychotherapist who can support the therapist in supporting the family.

In palliative care what is significant can seem comparatively small. Sometimes a parent can highlight the contribution of the occupational therapist. As one mother said after her daughter died, 'I'll never forget how you showed me to talk to June through my touch when her hearing and sight had gone. It meant so much to us both and I know that she knew I was there.' It is necessary that there is an opportunity for the occupational therapist to say 'goodbye' whether this is through reflective writing, attending the funeral, sending a card to the family and/or attending a prayer service. This allows for a sense of closure. Without it the occupational therapist and other staff will accumulate losses (Saunders and Valente, 1994) which can affect at an unconscious level and can lead to burnout.

SUMMARY

The occupational therapist can encounter a child referred for palliative care in the community, on an oncology ward, or at a hospice. The therapist may not be a specialist palliative care occupational therapist but will still need to adopt a palliative care approach. This means that occupational therapy and goal setting are still carried out but in a different way from curative therapy. It is important to remember that the whole family is supported in palliative care, and that the emotional as well as physical demands of a referred child or adolescent and their family are enormous. The pace of occupational therapy is different from a rehabilitative approach and the occupational therapist must adapt accordingly. This involves allocating more time when working with the child and family (Muhlenhaupt *et al.*, 1999).

It is helpful for the community occupational therapist to liaise with and get support from the specialist paediatric palliative care occupational therapist. The occupational therapist working with a child with a life-limiting condition needs support too. Working with babies, children and young adults in palliative care is demanding and challenging. This is a new and developing field for paediatric occupational therapists. The paediatric palliative care occupational therapist has a unique role and can make a positive contribution to the child and family and the multidisciplinary team at this very important stage in life.

ACTION POINTS

1. When is a child referred for palliative care?
2. How does a palliative occupational therapist's work differ from a community paediatric occupational therapist?

CASE STUDY

The occupational therapist is referred the following case. A single mother has an 8-year-old daughter who has an astrocytoma (brain tumour). The mother is losing sleep as her daughter is awake during the night. The daughter is struggling with her work at school and both are under emotional and physical strain. The child and her mother are referred to the children's hospice for respite breaks. The mother is reluctant to accept any help and battles on. The child's tumour grows and the child is now off her feet, at home all day and the mother has given up her work to care for her child full time. She contacts the hospice and asks for help. She says that she could not do this before as she felt she had to care for her child and might seem to be an 'inadequate mother' by asking for support.

In considering this family what would the occupational therapist involvement be, and which occupational therapy services would be involved?

REFERENCES

Addington-Hall, J. and Higginson, I. (2001) *Palliative Care for Non-Cancer Patients*, Oxford University Press, Oxford.

Bayley, N. (1993) *Bayley Scales of Infant Development*, The Psychological Corporation, San Antonio, TX.

Bion, W. R. (1984) *Learning From Experience*, Karnac Books, London.

Bowlby, J. (1988) *A Secure Base: Clinical applications of attachment theory*, Routledge, London.

Bray, J. and Cooper, J. (2004) The contribution to palliative medicine of allied health professions. *Oxford Textbook of Palliative Medicine*, 3rd edn (eds D. Doyle, G. Hanks, N. Cherny and K. Calman), Oxford University Press, Oxford.

Brown, C. (2001) Therapeutic play and creative arts. *Hospice Care for Children*, 2nd edn (eds A. Armstrong-Dailey and S. Zarbock), Oxford University Press, Oxford.

Case-Smith, J. (1998) *Pediatric Occupational Therapy and Early Intervention*, Butterworth-Heinemann, New York City, New York.

Cook, S. S., Renshaw, D. C. and Jackson, E. N. (1973) The dying child. *Occupational Therapy for Children* (ed. J. Case-Smith), Mosby, St Louis, MO.

Eland, J. M. (1981) Pain and symptom management. *Hospice Care for Children* (eds A. Armstrong-Dailey and S. Zarbock), Oxford University Press, Oxford.

Fraiberg, S. (1980) *Clinical Studies in Infant Mental Health*, Tavistock, London.

Frostig, M., Maslow, P., Lefever, D. W. and Whittlesey, J. R. B. (1963) *Frostig Developmental Test of Visual Perception*, Consulting Psychologists Press, Palo Alto, CA.

Gammage, S. H., McMahon, P. and Shanahan, P. (1976) Learning to cope with death. *American Journal of Occupational Therapy*, **30**(5), 294–9.

Goldman, A. and Schuller, I. (2001) Children and young adults, in *Palliative Care for Non-cancer Patients* (eds J. Addington-Hall and J. Higginson), Oxford University Press, Oxford.

Goodenough, F. F. and Harris, D. (1963) *The Goodenough-Harris Drawing Test*, The Psychological Corporation, London.

Grinyer, A. (2002) *Cancer in Young Adults*, Open University Press, Buckingham.

Henderson, S. E., Sugden, D. and Barnett, A. L. (1992) *Movement Assessment Battery for Children*, The Psychological Corporation, London.

Johnson-Soderberg, S. (1981) Children's concepts of death. *Oncology Nurses Forum*, **8**, 23–6.

Kew, S. (1975) *Handicap and Family Crisis*, Pitman Publishing, London.

Kielhofner, G. (2002) *A Model of Human Occupation: Theory and application*, Lippincott Williams & Wilkins, Philadelphia, PA.

Klein, M. (1998) *The Psycho-analysis of Children*, Karnac, London.

Kubler-Ross, E. (1969) *On Death and Dying*, Macmillan, New York.

Kubler-Ross, E. (1985) *On Children and Death*, Collier Books, New York.

Lansdown, R. (1987) The dying child's awareness of death. *Give Sorrow Words – Working with a Dying Child*, Whurr, London.

Lewin, J. and Reed, C. (1998) *Creative Problem Solving in Occupational Therapy*, Lippincott, USA.

Mosby, C. V. (1999) Foundations of pediatric practice. *Frames of Reference for Pediatric Occupational Therapy*, 2nd edn (eds P. Kramer and J. Hinojosa), Lippincott Williams & Wilkins, Philadelphia, PA.

Muhlenhaupt, M., Kramer, P. and Hinojosa, J. (1999) Perspective of context as related to frame of reference, in *Frames of Reference for Pediatric Occupational Therapy*, 2nd edn (eds P. Kramer and J. Hinojosa), Lippincott Williams & Wilkins, Philadelphia, PA.

Saunders, C. (1993) Foreword. *Oxford Textbook of Palliative Medicine* (eds D. Doyle, G. W. C. Hanks and N. MacDonald), Oxford University Press, Oxford.

Saunders, J. M. and Valente, S. M. (1994) Nurses' grief. *Cancer Nursing*, **17**(4), 318–25.

Sheridan, M. D. (2005) *From Birth to 5 Years*, The Children's Hospital, Sydney.

Wong, D. and Baker, C. (1988) Pain in children: A comparison of assessment scales. *Pediatric Nursing*, **4**(1), 9–17.

World Health Organization (1990) Cancer Pain Relief and Palliative Care Report *WHO Technical Report Series, No. 804*. Geneva: WHO.

SUGGESTED FURTHER READING

Ayres, J. (1991) *Sensory Integration and the Child*, Western Psychological Services, USA.

Bickerstaff, E. (1978) *Neurology*, Hodder & Stoughton, London.

Bowlby, J. (1997) *Attachment and Loss*, Pimlico, London.

Currer, C. (2001) *Responding to Grief – Dying, Bereavement and Social Care*, Palgrave, London.

Finnie, N. (1978) *Handling the Young Cerebral Palsied Child at Home*, Heinemann, London.

Harpin, P. (2000) *Adaptions Manual*, Muscular Dystrophy Campaign, London.

Hindmarch, C. (1993) *On The Death of a Child*, Radcliffe Medical Press, Oxford.

Jewett, C. (1994) *Helping Children Cope with Separation and Loss*, 2nd edn, Batsford, London.

Obholzer, A. and Zagier Roberts, V. (2002) *The Unconscious at Work*, Brunner-Routledge, London.

Sheridan, M. (1988) *From Birth to Five Years – Children's Developmental Progress*, NFER-Nelson, London.

Weininger, O. (1996) *Being and Not Being – Clinical Applications of the Death Instinct*, Karnac Books, London.

Winnicott, D. W. (1964) *The Child, the Family and the Outside World*, Penguin, London.

9 Occupational Therapy in HIV-related Cancers and Palliative Care

WILL CHEGWIDDEN AND CAMILLA HAWKINS

HIV AND AIDS

TRANSMISSION, PROGRESSION AND TREATMENT OF HIV

Human immunodeficiency virus (HIV) is a retrovirus which, if left untreated, replicates, thus depleting the immune system. This is evidenced clinically by a falling CD4 count and renders the person vulnerable to opportunistic infections. When healthy the individual's immune system is able to withstand and resist infection but through attacking CD4 cells HIV both destroys cells and causes them to become ineffective. HIV can also cause long-term damage to cells other than CD4 cells including certain type of neurones, and also plays a role in the development of certain types of cancers. HIV was first described in 1981 with effective treatments only becoming widely available in the mid-1990s. Prior to this many HIV-infected individuals progressed quickly to end stage disease. As such, research into the long-term effects of HIV and its link to neoplastic activity is relatively new.

Transmission of the virus can occur through unprotected oral, anal or vaginal sex, the transmission of blood and/or blood products (through needle sharing or non-sterile equipment and procedures), and vertical transmission (mother to child transmission [MTCT]) during pregnancy, delivery or breast feeding. The virus is present in varying concentrations in all body fluids. In the United Kingdom the most common transmission routes are far and away through unprotected sex. Whereas most new infections diagnosed in the UK in the 1980s and 1990s were via male-to-male sexual contact, since 1999 male-to-female and female-to-male sexual contact have been the most prevalent risk factor in new diagnoses, accounting for around 65% of all new recorded infections between 2002 and 2005 (Health Protection Agency, 2005). Although many of these infections were acquired outside of the UK and are linked to patterns of migration from sub-Saharan Africa,

Occupational Therapy in Oncology and Palliative Care. Edited by J. Cooper
© 2006 John Wiley & Sons Ltd

heterosexually-acquired HIV amongst British-born individuals is doubling every two to three years. Anonymous randomized testing also shows that around a quarter of all people with HIV are unaware of their status and remain untested (The UK Collaborative Group for HIV and STI Surveillance, 2004). Although vertical transmission is more prevalent in developing countries, the numbers of children diagnosed with HIV in the UK is relatively small, as are new diagnoses where the risk factor was sharing needles. Other risk factors are negligible in the UK, including occupational risks. Only five cases of occupationally acquired HIV have been recorded in the UK, out of 73 000 recorded HIV diagnoses (Tomkins and Ncube, 2005).

A diagnosis of acquired immune deficiency syndrome (AIDS) is given when a person's CD4 count falls below 200 and where they have been diagnosed with one or more from a standard list of opportunistic infections (OIs). Some clinics in the UK now shy away from using the term AIDS, as clinically it is less relevant now that there is not necessarily always a linear progression of disease, but rather episodic variations in health. The term AIDS also carries with it a degree of stigma. The Centre for Communicable Diseases (CCD) classification system (CCD A, B or C) is more often used to represent the degree of immunosuppression and the presence of more life-threatening conditions, with infected individuals able to move between the stages to reflect their state of HIV health (Fieldhouse, 2003).

Many classification systems exist for describing the symptoms, illnesses and conditions which are related to HIV. One way of dividing the illnesses is to consider illnesses and conditions in four broad categories.

- opportunistic infections are those which are allowed to occur to the body in an immunosupressed state;
- HIV-related malignancies are cancers which are either medically or statistically linked to HIV, but may occur when an individual is not necessarily significantly immunosupressed;
- auto-immune conditions are those that occur as a direct result of over-active and altered immune responses;
- constitutional conditions describe those that relate directly to the action of HIV on individual cells other than CD4 cells, including neurones and myocardial cells.

Table 9.1 summarizes these four categories and describes the underlying pathogenesis of the type of illness or condition.

One feature of HIV disease is that many of the illnesses and conditions listed above can affect more than one body system. For example, cytomegalovirus (CMV) infection can cause a retinitis that leads to eventual blindness, but can also infiltrate the gastrointestinal system leading to severe colitis, can cause lung disease, damage peripheral nerves, or cause central nervous system (CNS) impairment in either the brain or spinal cord. Many of the illnesses

Table 9.1 Categories and underlying pathogenesis in HIV/AIDS

Grouping	Action	Examples
Opportunistic infections (OIs)	These occur when an individual is immunosuppressed and thus has poor ability to avoid and fight infections. This is characterized by a low CD4 count.	• Viral infections including cytomegalovirus (CMV), progressive multifocal leukoencephalopathy (PML), herpes simplex virus (HSV) and varicella zoster virus (VZV); • Bacterial infections including tuberculosis (TB) and mycobacterium avium intracellulare (MAI); • Protozoal infections including toxoplasmosis and pneumocystis carinii pneumonia (PCP); • Fungal infections including cryptococcal meningitis and candida.
HIV-related malignancies	Not yet fully understood, however there is research that links certain precursor cells and viruses	• Non-Hodgkin's lymphoma including systemic NHL, primary central nervous system lymphoma and Burkitt's lymphoma; • Other lymphomas including Hodgkin's lymphoma; • Multicentric Castleman's disease; • Kaposi's sarcoma.
Auto-immune conditions	Complex patterns of immune system overactivity	• HIV-related arthralgia; • HIV-related Guillain-Barré syndrome; • Immune reconstitution illnesses – activation of other illnesses/OIs due to overactive immune response.
Constitutional	HIV affecting cells other than HIV cells	• Peripheral neuropathy where damage is caused to peripheral nerves by HIV itself; • HIV encephalopathy (HIVE); • AIDS dementia complex (ADC) – damage to central nervous system neurones by HIV itself; • Lipodystrophy, lipoatrophy, wasting syndromes, cardiac disease – some research implicates HIV itself affecting cells involved in cardiac function.

can cause CNS impairment. As some of the conditions and illnesses that cause CNS impairment cause global and others more focal damage, with varying response to treatment, presentations can vary widely from individual to individual.

It is important to be aware of the long latency period that can occur between infection and development of symptoms. During this time – which may be many years – the person may be asymptomatic and may have no reason to suspect health problems. Following transmission a seroconversion illness may be experienced where the person may feel unwell with a glandular fever or flu type illness which often is not attributed by the individual to HIV infection.

It is also important to consider the many variables that can influence patients' disease course, for example, the stage at which they present to healthcare services, the length of time that they have been HIV positive, other coexisting health and social care factors and the health and social care intervention that is available to them. Crucially, occupational therapists must take into account the context – environmental, financial, cultural, legal, social and geographical – within which the person functions – during all stages of assessment, intervention and planning.

The use of antiretroviral (ARV) medication can change the disease course, often dramatically. This has led to the disease being characterized as a chronic – but nevertheless still potentially life threatening – illness. This contrasts with the position in the first decade of the epidemic where a diagnosis of being HIV-positive was expected to lead automatically to an AIDS diagnosis and then to death, often within a short space of time. However, the possibilities offered by improved medical management of HIV exist primarily within western healthcare systems and the devastating impact of the pandemic, particularly in the African and Asian subcontinents, must not be underestimated (Fieldhouse, 2003).

CHANGING PRESENTATION OF PEOPLE LIVING WITH HIV AND AIDS (PLWHA)

Regionally within the UK, London and the South East remain the areas of highest number of PLWHA per capita and in absolute numbers, and the primary focus of many HIV services and organizations. Despite this, all UK regions have seen increases in new diagnoses since 1999, with a growing trend for new HIV infection and new AIDS diagnosis to be reported at the same time. In some areas previously of low prevalence, rates of new diagnoses have more than doubled (Health Protection Agency, 2005).

Overall, an increasingly diverse group of individuals is affected, both in terms of a widening age spectrum, social and cultural background and lifestyle. This can have widespread implications for occupational therapy intervention. Individuals may be older and affected by age-related illnesses, or may have coexisting physical or mental health diagnoses which influence the management of their HIV health.

A proportion of individuals are presenting late to health services. This may limit their treatment options, as their immune systems will have already been compromised. They may be unaware that they have been at risk or be concerned about presenting to formal, statutory services, for example, if they have immigration or other legal issues.

Antiretroviral medication, which has become widely available in the UK since the mid-1990s, has led to dramatically increased life expectancies, and this, coupled with improvements in the treatment of HIV-associated illnesses and conditions and improvements in prophylactic treatment (which prevent reoccurrence of these conditions), has led to a change in the range of commonly seen illnesses and presentations. Once common, life-threatening illnesses such as PML and Kaposi's sarcoma are now see far less commonly, and others such as PCP are treated far more effectively and benefit from improved prophylactic treatment. However, rates of TB infection and cardiac disease have surged in recent years.

CHANGING ROLE OF OCCUPATIONAL THERAPY WITH PLWHA

The role of the occupational therapist with PLWHA has altered in line with the changing presentations of PLWHA. Short- and medium-term interventions, often with a focus on palliative and end-of-life issues, have given way to a chronic disease management model focusing on living well and long-term lifestyle management. In the acute and rehabilitation setting, the focus is far more on rehabilitation and community reintegration rather than palliation and respite. Occupational therapists are beginning to work with teenagers who have been HIV-positive since birth and are making life goals and choices around work, study and relationships. There is an emerging role for occupational therapists to be involved with vocational services for PLWHA. If one thing characterizes therapists working with an HIV-positive population it is that they are likely to encounter individuals at very different stages of the journey through their illness with a wide variety of needs, goals and circumstances.

Occupational therapy practice with PLWHA may encompass many of the following aspects:

Functional/physical care

- assessment of physical function and personal and domestic activities of daily living, in the context of the individual's goals, taking account of any physical or cognitive deficit as well as the potential impact of psychological aspects such as low mood, decreased motivation or initiation, placing this in the context of their home environment and statutory or non-statutory support as well as longer term prognosis;

- where appropriate, adoption of a compensatory approach by teaching an alternative technique or method of performing a task or investigating provision of equipment. Key issues are looking at energy conservation, task simplification and adaptation of the environment to promote safety and independence. Liaison with community social care services regarding packages of care;
- where appropriate, adoption of a rehabilitative approach to improve strength, endurance, praxis/coordination or other aspects of physical function;
- awareness of the impact that multiple pathologies may have and adoption of mixed methods as appropriate; for example, a rehabilitative approach may help address an underlying weakness secondary to recovering respiratory function whereas a concurrent persistent unilateral neurological upper limb weakness may require compensatory equipment, adaptations or assistance.

Psychological and social care

- identification of stressors and their role in the maintenance of a healthy immune system;
- assessment, advice and information on stress management including relaxation techniques;
- identification of new or pre-existing mental health issues that may be reactive to coming to terms with an HIV diagnosis, or related to a diagnosable psychological manifestation of an HIV-CNS impairment including mania, psychosis, depression or psychomotor symptoms;
- practical issues such as housing and financial issues need to be addressed. As many people in the UK with an HIV diagnosis have arrived from other countries and may not have legal status in the UK, many may be living in unsuitable and overcrowded conditions, may have no home at all, and no recourse to public housing or public funds. There is a significant incidence of breakdown of primary supports at time of diagnosis (partner, family, friends) for many individuals and working with the multidisciplinary team and community resources to solve these practical issues is often necessary before other rehabilitative or emotional goals can be addressed;
- awareness that some PLWHA have come from countries where they have escaped war and possibly torture and the impact of this on their mental health. Others may have escaped countries where their sexuality may have also led to persecution.

HIV-related brain impairment and cognitive assessment and rehabilitation

Occupational therapists need to provide formal cognitive assessment to give information on a range of cognitive skills, such as orientation, memory, comprehension or problem solving. This informs input with the individual in terms of strengths, needs, abilities and avenues for meaningful activity and occupation. Occupational therapists should be aware that this area of brain impairment, in terms of prognosis and the demographics of the population, is relatively new and not yet well researched. This means that therapists may be utilizing assessments that may not be standardized for the specific client group and therefore results must be interpreted accordingly.

Individuals should be empowered wherever possible regarding participation in decision making, planning and producing ideas for activities and interventions. This collaboration recognizes the person's skills and abilities and promotes cooperation and engagement. Group work is often used very successfully in slow-stream cognitive rehabilitation, and can include focused, process work groups, functional tasks and community and social tasks. The demographic of an HIV population in the UK often means that activities that therapists would commonly undertake in a cognitive rehabilitation setting may be of less relevance or require considerable modification. The therapist needs to be acutely aware of the group members' backgrounds and preferences. Memory is often an area that therapists become involved with assessing and treating, including developing external cues and prompts, although it is vital to recognize that there may be a point where, even when making use of information; equipment and adaptations, an individual is unable to continue to be safe and independent and requires assistance from a carer, formal or informal.

The role of occupational therapists in assessing and providing intervention related to activities of daily living should not be underestimated as it is particularly important when planning for future discharge. There are frequently complex housing, social, physical and psychological needs and these will need to be assessed and intervention focused on maximizing independence and function while promoting safety. Liaison with a variety of professionals and agencies is usually necessary to ensure a suitable and comprehensive care package. The multidisciplinary team remains paramount in managing the often complex and multidimensional needs of an individual with HIV.

HIV-RELATED CANCERS

This section discusses the incidence and presentation of cancers that are related to or more commonly seen in individuals with HIV infection.

RESEARCH

A number of cancers occur more frequently in an HIV-positive population than in the general population, with 30–40% of all PLWHA experiencing some kind of a malignancy in their lifetime. For HIV-positive people, the likelihood that they will develop a cancer in comparison to non-HIV infected individuals varies between two- to three-fold for some cancers up to over one hundred times or more likely for others (Newcomb-Fernandez, 2003). The exact relationship between HIV and neoplastic activity is not fully understood, although a range of other normally relatively harmless viruses have been implicated in having some kind of causative or catalyst role. This is discussed in more detail later in this section.

Although low CD4 counts correlate with higher rates of malignancy, malignancies still occur in individuals with comparatively high CD4 counts, in contrast to other opportunistic infections that occur only when CD4 counts are low. Since the advent of HAART (highly active antiretroviral therapy) malignancies have risen from being the cause of death in 10–15% of HIV-positive individuals to over one quarter (Bonnet et al., 2004). It is not clear why this is so although it is postulated that there may be some relationship between long-term HIV infection and the risk of abnormal cell behaviour that precipitates the development of some malignancies (Newcomb-Fernandez, 2003; Killebrew and Shiramizu, 2004). Some of the otherwise relatively harmless viruses that have been linked to cancers in HIV-infected individuals include:

Table 9.2 HIV-related cancers

Virus	Linked with the development of
Human herpes virus 8 (HHV-8)	Kaposi's sarcoma
Human papilloma virus (HPV)	Anal and cervical cancer
Epstein-Barr virus (EBV)	Lymphoma
Hepatitis B and C viruses (HBV and HPC)	Liver cancer

(Adapted from Gadd (ed.) 2005)

Some of the more common cancers seen in HIV are Kaposi's sarcoma, primary CNS lymphoma, Hodgkin's lymphoma, anal cancer and Burkitt's lymphoma. It is worth noting that some common epithelial cancers such as breast, prostate and colon cancer do not occur more commonly in an HIV-infected population (Cheung, 2005; Pantanowitz and Dezube, 2005).

Outside of countries where advanced treatment is widely available, and in particular in sub-Saharan Africa where over half the world's HIV-positive population lives, malignancies commonly seen in resource-rich countries in HIV-positive populations in the pre-HAART era, such as Kaposi's sarcoma and non-Hodgkin's lymphoma, are still increasing in incidence. However, Hodgkin's disease does not appear to have become more prevalent (Orem, Otieno and Remick, 2004).

Treatments for cancers in PLWHA often are similar to those in a non-infected individual, although some modifications may need to be made dependent on the underlying state of HIV health and possible drug interactions. Improvements in HAART mean that survival duration statistics are approaching those seen in HIV-negative individuals, although the statistics are not consistent across all cancers (Thirwell et al., 2003).

NON-HODGKIN'S LYMPHOMA (NHL)

This is one of the most long-associated malignancies with HIV, having first been described in 1982. Most NHLs are B-cell in origin, with most of these being either a diffuse large-cell B-cell lymphoma or a Burkitt's lymphoma. A small number are primary effusion lymphomas (PELs). When the primary site of the NHL is in the CNS, it is known as a primary CNS lymphoma (PCNSL), otherwise it is generally classified as systemic NHL (Hoffman and Kamps, 2003; Gadd, 2005).

Systemic NHLs tend to present as lymph node enlargement, with often a systemic extranodal focus, in any body region. The disease is often aggressive and although treatment has improved in the era of HAART, average prognosis still remains at around two years. Secondary CNS involvement is common. As there are drug interactions between antiretroviral therapy and conventional NHL treatments, the treatment protocol for NHLs in PLWHA is still considered experimental. Some researchers and clinicians advocate an interruption to ARV treatment to maximize the response to chemotherapy, seeing the NHL treatment as the priority; others advocate no interruption to HIV treatment (Aboulafia, Pantanowitz and Dezube, 2004; Gadd, 2005).

PRIMARY CNS LYMPHOMA (PCNSL)

PCNSL was previously a major cause of death in HIV-infected individuals with a prevalence of up to 10% and poor average prognosis of only a few months from diagnosis. Since the advent of HAART the incidence has decreased considerably and mean survival time has increased to up to two years (Hoffman and Kamps, 2003). PCNSL is almost always associated with the presence of Epstein-Barr virus (EBV) in HIV-infected individuals. Obtaining a differential diagnosis from other CNS pathology can be difficult; especially obtaining a differential diagnosis from the most common cerebral mass lesion, cerebral toxoplasmosis (Newell *et al.*, 2004). PCNSL is more likely to be a solitary mass than cerebral toxoplasmosis, although there may be two to four lesions. On CT scan lesions are usually enhancing with variable oedema. Frontal lobe lesions are most common, and lesions may cross the midline. Common presentations include confusion, personality changes, focal deficits, headaches and seizure activity (Brew, 2001; Hoffman and Kamps, 2003; Newell *et al.*, 2004). Treatment is not yet well defined and may include radiation, chemotherapy, HAART and treatment of the associated EBV. Current research results from multi-centre trials indicate that in future improved survival and long-term neurologic function in patients with PCNSL is likely (Batara and Grossman, 2003). This may mean for therapists that these patients will be on the whole more appropriate for active rehabilitation rather than palliation as treatment options improve.

BURKITT'S LYMPHOMA

Unlike other common HIV-related NHLs, the incidence of Burkitt's lymphoma has not decreased in the era of HAART. Burkitt's lymphoma in HIV-positive individuals may be the same as a classic Burkitt's lymphoma or may have a plasmacytoid differentiation only seen in HIV. Peripheral blood and bone marrow are often involved (Newcomb-Fernandez, 2003; Aboulafia, Pantanowitz and Dezube, 2004). The outcome is generally poor and poor outcome closely correlates with low CD4 counts (Gadd, 2005).

PRIMARY EFFUSION LYMPHOMA (PEL)

This is a rare form of NHL also known as 'body cavity-based lymphoma' and primarily seen in HIV populations. It is characterized by body cavity effusions in pleural and pericardial cavities, and ascites. PEL is aggressive, the outcome is generally poor and treatments experimental (Newcomb-Fernandez, 2003; Aboulafia, Pantanowitz and Dezube, 2004; Gadd, 2005).

HODGKIN'S DISEASE (HD)

Hodgkin's disease is a type of lymphoma found both in the general population and in HIV-positive populations. Incidence is higher in HIV-positive populations, although not greatly so. In HIV-negative populations HD tends to present earlier, is less aggressive and generally considered a treatable tumour. In contrast, HD in people with HIV is often aggressive, more likely to spread from the lymphatic system to other sites and mean prognosis is poor. HD is characterized by a Pel-Ebstein rising and falling fever, anaemia and weakness. Treatment in early stages is usually radiotherapy with chemotherapy being adopted in later stages (Hoffman and Kamps, 2003; Gadd, 2005; Lim and Levine, 2005).

KAPOSI'S SARCOMA

Kaposi's sarcoma (KS) is a common malignancy in HIV-positive populations and primarily presents as skin lesions, although it can also have visceral, oral, gastrointestinal (GI) or pulmonary manifestations. It was the emergence of KS amongst young gay men in San Francisco and New York in 1981 that partially lead to the identification of HIV as a new disease. In early stages KS tends to present as purplish-black lesions that may appear anywhere on the body. Treatment in early stages is with HAART to address underlying immunosuppression; chemotherapy and local therapies may be indicated in more advanced disease (Krown, 2003; Casper, 2004).

Mucous membrane and visceral complications may occur with skin lesions or independently. Mild cases of skin lesions that are neither painful nor restrict function may not be treated and patients may be given advice on camouflaging lesions until they resolve. As skin lesions may occur anywhere, they can lead to functional problems, for example, lesions on the foreskin or glans penis may cause difficulty managing urination. GI Kaposi's sarcoma is often asymptomatic but may lead to pain or bleeding. Oral lesions may cause difficulty with eating and speaking. Most serious is pulmonary KS and this can be fatal, particularly as it is more prevalent in patients with advanced HIV disease (Krown, 2003; Gadd, 2005).

Until the advent of HIV, Kaposi's sarcoma was rare and occurred in various forms in older Mediterranean men, African children and people who had been treated with immunosuppressive drugs. The epidemic form of KS, which is the form associated with HIV, is thought to be linked to the HHV-8 virus, which is sexually transmitted. HIV-associated KS varies widely in extent and aggression of the disease process. Since the advent of HAART, Kaposi's sarcoma is far less prevalent in countries where antiretroviral medication is widely available. In the rest of the world, KS remains a significant problem (Orem, Otieno and Remick, 2004; Gadd, 2005).

The role of the therapist with individuals with HIV-related KS depends on the extent of the disease and the nature of any functional or cosmetic impairment. For people with advanced disease a palliative approach may be appropriate; with recovering pulmonary disease a rehabilitative approach may be indicated; for skin lesions causing functional problems novel problem solving may be required.

MULTI-CENTRIC CASTLEMAN'S DISEASE (MCD) AND CASTLEMAN'S SYNDROME

These relatively rare and poorly understood lymphoproliferative disorders are associated with the human herpes virus (HHV-8) and Kaposi's sarcoma. Hepatomegaly, anaemia and respiratory symptoms are common; MCD appears to lead to NHL in many instances, thus rendering the outcome of MCD often poor. Treatment may be chemotherapy and splenectomy in advanced disease (Hoffman and Kamps, 2003; Gadd, 2005).

OTHER HIV-RELATED CANCERS

LUNG CANCER

Although there is some variation in the literature, in the UK the rate of lung cancer amongst HIV-positive individuals is much higher than in the general population. Although there may be some links to non-HIV related well-proven risks (e.g. higher rates of smoking amongst young gay and bisexual men), there have also been observed differences in the histological presentation, age at presentation and progression of the disease, and low CD4 count has also been linked with higher incidence of lung cancer. This would all suggest there is some link between lung cancer and HIV that is not yet fully understood. The assumption that HAART may result in the increased risk of malignancy may explain the link to the higher incidence of lung cancer (Northfelt, 2003; Gadd, 2005; Lim and Levine, 2005).

ANO-RECTAL CANCERS

Studies demonstrate that people with HIV are between 30 and 50 times more likely to develop an anal carcinoma than HIV-negative individuals. A link between these carcinomas and the human papillomavirus (HPV) has been established, although no correlation between levels of immunosuppression and incidence of anal cancer has been shown. Outcomes are often poor in HIV-infected individuals. Rates are higher amongst gay and bisexual men; however, a history of anal sex is no longer implicated as being a predisposing factor in the presence of HPV or the development of an anal carcinoma (Newcomb-Fernandez, 2003; Lim and Levine, 2005).

CERVICAL CANCER

Although cervical cancer is listed on the CDC stages B and C as defining ill-nesses, the relationship between invasive cervical cancer (ICC) and HIV is somewhat inconsistent in the literature. As with anal carcinomas, there is a strong link between HPV and the development of ICC (Newcomb-Fernandez, 2003).

MULTIPLE MYELOMA

Evidence is emerging that plasma cell neoplasms are being reported with increasing incidence within HIV-positive populations, and that multiple myelomas (MMs) have features that differentiate it from MMs in non-HIV populations. At present treatment remains as for MM in non-HIV popula-tions (Cheung, 2005; Pantanowitz and Dezube, 2005).

OTHER CANCERS

Some other cancers do appear to have a slightly to moderately increased incidence within HIV populations although in some instances other factors such as smoking rates, gender and ageing populations may have an impact. Cancers that have been described as having increased incidence within an HIV-positive population include leiomyosarcoma, germ cell malignancies, non-melanoma skin cancers and a range of systemic cancers e.g. stomach, liver, kidney. More research is required with these conditions (Newcomb-Fernandez, 2003; Northfelt, 2003).

OTHER HIV-RELATED LIFE-LIMITING CONDITIONS

The mortality rate has dropped dramatically since the introduction of HAART in the UK, although the number of deaths secondary to HIV remains significant at over 500 per year (Health Protection Agency, 2005).

The nature of the HIV-related illness or condition(s) that eventually lead to death has also changed since the advent of HAART. There is a much lower incidence of diseases overall that cause a gradual decline, where the occupational therapist and the multidisciplinary team are involved in planning for end stage disease. Many of the deaths reported in London HIV services are as a result of acute illnesses, where the patient is being treated acutely and aggressively for one or more major HIV-related illness or conditions, often in an intensive treatment setting where therapist input is not appropriate and a palliative approach is not taken until the very last hours or days of illness, or not at all should an acute event such as multi-organ failure, myocardial infarction or massive neurological event suddenly occur. Patients who present to hospital with late stage HIV disease may have multiple HIV-related pathologies, very poor immune systems/CD4 counts and co-existent health problems such as TB. These patients tend to die in the acute phase of their treatment or recover and require a rehabilitative approach, rather than progress to requiring terminal care from the multidisciplinary team.

Given the potential complex medical presentation of some patients with late stage HIV disease, and the relative newness of HIV as a condition, some patients' acute illness remain undiagnosed until death and post mortem. Without a diagnosis medical teams (and often patients and families) are often reluctant to move to a palliative model of care and instead favour aggressive treatment.

Apart from the malignancies described earlier in this chapter, the two other HIV-related illnesses that tend to require a palliative approach are PML (progressive multifocal leukoencephalopathy) and HIV encephalopathy/AIDS dementia complex/HIV associated dementia (HIVE/ADC/HAD). There is no specific effective direct treatment for any these conditions and neurological recovery occurs as immune system repair occurs secondary to HAART. Where significant repair is not possible and a patient is not responding virologically due to the development of drug resistance or the presence of very advanced disease, a palliative approach may be adopted by the team. Common presentations for these conditions include deteriorating cognitive function, behaviour and personality changes, and focal neurology including

paresis or weakness. Severe and life-limiting forms of both PML and HIVE/
HAD are considerably more rare than in the era before HAART (Gadd,
2005).

HIV AND PALLIATIVE CARE

A number of factors in HIV service provision have resulted, in some instances,
in an inequality in accessing quality palliative care services, both in terms of
end-of-life care and access to good pain and symptom control. Some of the
main complicating factors include:

- disease factors such as lack of predictability of a course of disease and
  the complexity of treatments;
- demographic factors including the impact of poverty, homelessness, concurrent intravenous drug use, chaotic lifestyles and language/cultural
  issues;
- service factors such as inappropriate curative focus and stigma and discrimination from mainstream services.

(Harding, Easterbrook, Higginson *et al.*, 2005)

The scope of this chapter does not allow for a full discussion of all of these
factors, however some of the major themes are identified as follows:

GUILT, STIGMA AND ATTITUDES TO DEATH AND DYING –
ISSUES FOR PEOPLE COMING TO THE UK

For individuals who originally came from outside the UK, there may be
myriad causes for feelings of stress, stigma, guilt and anger. They may originally have entered the UK on a work or student visa. Through illness they
may be unable to continue in their intended study or work role. This can have
consequences for their financial situation, housing, future role and expectations. Frequently, individuals are responsible for an extended family in their
country of origin and if they are unable to fulfil expectations, the strain can
be immense. They may have had plans of bringing their children and partners
or spouses to the UK or of returning to their home country with additional
qualifications or skills that would improve their financial standing and ability
to support others. Such plans are likely to be disrupted, perhaps only tempo-
rarily, or perhaps for many years if immigration and legal issues need to be
explored and addressed. Many people have come from communities where
death from HIV has been prevalent and the disease very stigmatized. Misin-
formation on transmission, prognosis and treatment options, propagated in
their home countries, communities and sometimes by churches to which they
belong, can intensify feelings of guilt and isolation.

ISSUES FOR GAY MEN, BISEXUAL MEN, AND OTHER MEN WHO HAVE SEX WITH MEN

Although considerable progress has been made since the early eighties within the gay and bisexual community with relation to sexuality and the acceptance of HIV-diagnosed people on both an individual and organizational basis, examples of stigma and discrimination still remain. In addition to dealing with a new HIV diagnosis or a deteriorating illness, individuals may feel unable to be open about their sexuality and/or their HIV status with partners, family, friends and work colleagues. This can lead to relationship breakdown and loss of social support, and these issues may be intensified in an end-of-life situation. For men who have little support within or little access to the resources within the gay and bisexual community, and for men who have sex with men but don't identify with being gay or bisexual, feelings of guilt and isolation can also be considerable, and complicated by lack of access to information and support. Actual episodes of homophobic abuse still occur, and often are more prevalent and go unreported outside of major centres.

ACCESS TO MAINSTREAM SERVICES

Access to mainstream services, such as social services care and equipment services, hospices and non-HIV-specific health and pain management services, may be affected by real or perceived discrimination on the grounds of HIV status, HIV status and sexuality, or HIV status and lifestyle factors such as being a known drug user or commercial sex worker. There is evidence that some hospice staff are uncomfortable working with HIV-positive patients, and anecdotal evidence that in settings outside of large cities, local clinics and services do not always respond with the same level of sensitivity compared with diverse metropolitan areas (Harding *et al.*, 2005).

THE IMPACT OF UNCERTAIN DISEASE PROGRESSION

Unlike many other deteriorating conditions, the unpredictable and non-linear nature of HIV disease since the advent of antiretroviral therapy has led to a situation where individuals are faced with a constant level of uncertainty. Individuals with advanced HIV may develop a life-threatening illness, then recover, and then develop another life-threatening illness, and so on. Elevated levels of health-related anxiety mean that common non-specific symptoms may take on an increased level of significance and individuals may find their ability to formulate long-term goals impaired. It is questionable whether the current presentation of HIV fits with a traditional palliative care paradigm (Cochrane, 2003).

MEDICATION, ADHERENCE AND PAIN MANAGEMENT ISSUES

MEDICATION, SIDE-EFFECTS AND ADHERENCE

In the UK, statistics show a sharp initial drop in the rate of disease progression in 1997, followed by a more moderate but significant linear decline to 2001. This reflects the widespread use of antiretroviral therapy at this time. Individuals were finding that even where they had a very low CD4, medical intervention through ARV therapy could result in dramatic clinical recovery and increased life expectancy.

The decision of whether or not to commence treatment may be recommended by the medical team due to the person having a low CD4 count (in the UK treatment is recommended when the CD4 count is between 200 and 350) (Gazzard, 2005). Commencing antiretroviral therapy may prevent opportunistic infections – through inhibiting the replication of the virus – or may benefit the person in terms of controlling existing illnesses and symptoms.

However, medication should not be viewed as a panacea, since aside from the social, cultural and environmental influences that may impair adherence, the medication itself may cause side-effects. For those who have not experienced side-effects from the HIV disease process itself, to experience them from the medication is especially challenging and is an indicator for reduced adherence. Naturally, the medical team will attempt to minimize any side-effects through the use of anti-emetics, anti-diarrhoeals, etc. Research and development by drug manufacturers attempts to address such issues as pill burden (number of tablets), unpalatability, size of tablets, and stipulations of certain regimes such as diet and timing. New advances are constantly occurring, and although this offers the potential for future improvements, it can also lead to a perception by some individuals that they do not need to consider the potential consequences of risky behaviour since medication is available.

In order for medication benefits to be optimized it is necessary for adherence to be above 95% and this relates to the timing of the doses as well as the actual number of doses. Fitting the doses into other daily routines such as work, caring for dependants or children, can be problematic, particularly where others in the person's life may be unaware of their HIV status. Additionally there can be significant problems where there are alcohol and substance issues. Not only can these negatively impact upon adherence but may also lead to specific health problems in their own right, for example, where someone has binges, engages in risky behaviour due to lowered inhibition or awareness and/or loses track of time and consequently cannot keep to a regular routine.

Individuals may dislike the daily psychological reminder of their diagnosis that medication can provide. Additionally, even when established successfully on a regime, there may be a psychological burden of uncertainty and fear for the future in terms of continued control of their illness, or the possibility of a deterioration or difficulty.

For individuals with unresolved immigration status, being placed in multiple occupancy accommodation or without adequate refrigeration and other storage facilities may affect their ability to maintain confidentiality and safe storage, which can impact upon adherence and effectiveness of ARV regimes. Some individuals face the threat of deportation to countries where medication is neither affordable nor accessible to them geographically, despite official sources stating that effective ARV medications are available.

PAIN AND SYMPTOM MANAGEMENT

Pain and symptom control is a major issue for many HIV-positive people. Pain may be secondary to a number of the illnesses and conditions listed above, and include painful peripheral neuropathies, which may be a side-effect of medication, a direct consequence of HIV on peripheral nerves, or part of an opportunistic infection, e.g. Guillain-Barré syndrome.

Occupational therapists can play an important role in the multidisciplinary assessment and treatment of pain, including advice and information around managing types of pain, relaxation techniques, energy conservation and provision of adaptive techniques and equipment.

FUTURE CHALLENGES FOR OCCUPATIONAL THERAPY

Within a western healthcare context, the extended life expectancy and potential opportunities for maintaining physical, psychological and cognitive health and function will enable many individuals with HIV to engage in a wide range of activities and occupational roles. People may choose to explore training, paid employment or a return to education. They may also feel they have the freedom to make choices in their personal life, such as having children, travelling, and developing relationships. The uncertain nature of the relationship of some cancers with HIV and the dual factors of (a) increasing prevalence of some HIV-related cancers and (b) increasing survival rates and/or times, means that therapists are likely to be treating more and more people with both diagnoses. These patients are likely to have complex medical and social backgrounds and often uncertain futures. Flexibility of approach while remaining person- and occupation-centred will continue to be a challenge for therapists working with these individuals. Although a palliative approach will still be indicated for a smaller number of individuals, perhaps many more may find issues of managing chronic illness and addressing occupational roles and vocational needs will be the key components of a successful and person-centred therapeutic approach. Developing an evidence base that keeps pace with medical advances and changes in presentation will continue to present a challenge to therapists.

REFERENCES

Aboulafia, D. M., Pantanowitz, L. and Dezube, B. J. (2004) AIDS-related non-Hodgkin lymphoma: Still a problem in the era of HAART. *AIDS Reader*, **14**(11), 605–17.

Batara, J. F. and Grossman, S. A. (2003) Primary central nervous system lymphomas. *Current Opinion in Neurology*, **16**, 671–5.

Bonnet, F., Lewden, C., May, D., Heripret, L., Jougla, E., Costagliola, D., *et al.* (2004) Malignancies-related causes of death of HIV-infected patients in the era of highly active antiretroviral therapy. Poster presentation at *11th Conference on Retroviruses and Opportunistic Infections* Feb 8–11, 2004. San Francisco.

Brew, B. J. (2001) *HIV Neurology*, Oxford University Press, Sydney.

Casper, C. (2004) Human Herpesvirus-8, Kaposi Sarcoma and AIDS-associated neoplasms. *HIV InSite Knowledge Base Chapter*. Accessed online 06.07.2005 at http://hivinsite.ucsd.edu

Cheung, M. C. (2005) AIDS-related malignancies: Emerging challenges in the era of highly active antiretroviral therapy. *The Oncologist*, **10**(6), 412–26.

Cochrane, J. (2003) The experience of uncertainty for individuals with HIV/AIDS and the palliative care paradigm. *International Journal of Palliative Nursing*, **9**(9), 382–8.

*Fieldhouse, R. (ed.) (2003) *Aids Reference Manual*, National AIDS Manual, London.

*Gadd, C. (ed.) (2005) *National AIDS Manual: HIV and AIDS Treatments Directory*, 24th edn, National AIDS Manual, London.

Gazzard, B. on behalf of the BHIVA Writing Committee (2005) British HIV Association (BHIVA) guidelines for the treatment of HIV infected adults with antiretroviral therapy – 2005. *HIV Medicine*, **6**(S2), 1–61.

Harding, R., Easterbrook, P., Higginson, I. J., Karus, D., Raveis, V. H. and Marconi, K. (2005) Access and equity in HIV/AIDS palliative care: A review of the evidence and responses. *Palliative Medicine*, **19**, 251–8.

Health Protection Agency (2005) *AIDS/HIV Quarterly Surveillance Tables: Cumulative data to end June 2005*, Health Protection Agency and the Scottish Centre For Infection and Environmental Health and the Institute of Child Health, London.

Hoffman, C. and Kamps, B. S. (2003) *HIV Medicine 2003*. Accessed online 06.07.2005 at http://www.hivmedicine.com/pdf/hivmedicine2003.pdf

Killebrew, D. and Shiramizu, B. (2004) Pathogenesis of HIV-associated non-Hodgkin lymphoma. *Current HIV Research*, **2**(3), 215–21.

Krown, S. E. (2003) Clinical characteristics of Kaposi Sarcoma. *HIV InSite Knowledge Base Chapter*. Accessed online 06.07.2005 at http://hivinsite.ucsd.edu

Lim, S. T. and Levine, A. M. (2005) Non-AIDS-defining cancers and HIV infection. *Current Infectious Diseases Reports*, **7**, 227–34.

Newell, M. E., Hoy, J. F., Cooper, S. G., DeGraaff, B., Grulich, A. E. and Bryant, M. (2004) Human Immunodeficiency Virus-related primary central nervous system lymphoma: Factors influencing survival in 111 patients. *Cancer*, **100**(12), 2627–36.

Newcomb-Fernandez, J. (2003) Data review: Cancer in the HIV-infected population. *Research Initiative Treatment Action*, **9**(1). Accessed online 06.07.2005 www.centerforaods.org/rita/0903/epi.htm

Northfelt, D. W. (2003) Other malignancies associated with HIV. *HIV InSite Knowledge Base Chapter.* Accessed online 06.07.2005 at http://hivinsite.ucsd.edu

Orem, J., Otieno, M. W. and Remick, S. (2004) AIDS-associated cancer in developing nations. *Current Opinion in Neuology,* **16,** 468–76.

Pantanowitz, L. and Dezube, B. J. (2005) AIDS-related cancer: New entities, emerging targets, and novel tactics. *Haematological Oncology,* **8**(1), 20–30.

Thirwell, C., Sarker, S., Stebbing, J. and Bower, M. (2003) Acquired immunodeficiency related lymphoma in the era of highly active antiretroviral therapy. *Clinical Lymphoma,* **4**(2), 86–92.

Tomkins, S. and Ncube, F. (2005) *Occupational Transmission of HIV: Summary of published reports, March 2005 edition,* Health Protection Agency and Collaborators, London.

The UK Collaborative Group for HIV and STI Surveillance (2004) *Focus on Prevention: HIV and other sexually transmitted infections in the United Kingdom in 2003,* Health Protection Agency Centre for Infections, London.

*Recommended reading/reference.

Note: The information published in the regularly updated National AIDS Manual publications are also available online at www.aidsmap.co.uk. The site is regularly updated with information, research and developments and is aimed both at HIV-positive people and health and social care professionals. The *AIDS Reference Manual* is a thorough resource on the social impact of HIV and AIDS and includes information on the origins of the epidemic, transmission, testing, prevention, vaccines and the law, as well as information on living well with HIV, caring for someone with HIV and working with children and families affected by HIV. The *HIV and AIDS Treatment Directory* is a comprehensive guide to medical aspects of HIV and AIDS including an A–Z listing of symptoms, illnesses, treatments and medical tests, and chapters covering the immune system, HIV lifecycle, and drugs used by people with HIV.

10 Occupational Therapy in Neuro-oncology

HELEN BARRETT AND JULIE WATTERSON

CENTRAL NERVOUS SYSTEM TUMOURS

Brain and spinal cord tumours, collectively known as central nervous system (CNS) tumours, occur as a result of abnormal cell growth inside the skull or spinal column. Malignant primary brain tumours can grow quickly and spread to other areas of the brain but will rarely spread to other parts of the body. Benign CNS tumours grow relatively slowly and are usually confined to one location. Benign tumours can potentially be harmful as any growth within the confined space of the skull or spinal column can place pressure on sensitive tissues and consequently have an impact on function.

The causes of CNS tumours are largely unknown but in a small number of individuals they may result from specific genetic diseases, such as neurofibromatosis, immune system disorders (e.g. HIV) or exposure to radiation or carcinogenic chemicals.

Brain tumours can occur at any age but are more common in adults over 45 years of age. They account for around 2% of all cancers (Soo *et al.*, 1997). Each year in the UK there are approximately 2500 new cases of brain tumours in men and 1800 in women (Cancer Research UK, 2005). 10–30% of adults with cancer develop brain metastases, which are the most common type of brain tumour in adults (Wen and Loeffler, 1999). Brain metastases are usually multiple, with the lung and breast being the most common primary sites. Spinal cord tumours are less common than brain tumours and can affect people of all ages, though are more prevalent in young and middle-aged adults.

CLASSIFICATIONS

Brain tumours are classified according to the cells where they originate (e.g. gliomas from glial cells, astrocytomas from astrocytes). The World Health

Occupational Therapy in Oncology and Palliative Care. Edited by J. Cooper
© 2006 John Wiley & Sons Ltd

Organization classifies over 80 sub-types of brain tumours (Kleihues *et al.*, 1993). The most common primary brain tumours are gliomas, which account for approximately half of all brain tumours. Gliomas are further classified according to the type of glial cell involved. Gliomas are also categorized by histology and the differentiation of cells; high-grade tumours are poorly differentiated and fast growing and low-grade are well differentiated and tend to be slow growing. Low-grade gliomas are likely to transform into high-grade tumours. Typically an individual with a low-grade glioma can anticipate on average a prognosis of up to 10 years. The prognosis for someone with a glioblastoma multiforme (GBM), a high grade tumour, is 12 to 18 months from diagnosis (Hill *et al.*, 2002). Spinal cord tumours are divided into extra-dural and intradural (which are subdivided into extramedullary and intramedullary).

SIGNS AND SYMPTOMS

CNS tumours can cause a number of signs and symptoms depending on the size, type and location. Most common are:

- headaches
- seizures
- poor coordination and balance
- hemiparesis/hemiplegia
- weakness (focal or global)
- sensory disturbances (e.g. blurred or double vision, numbness or altered sensation in upper and/or lower limbs)
- cognitive deficits (e.g. confusion, memory deficits)
- personality and behavioural changes
- drowsiness and lethargy
- difficulty swallowing
- slurring of speech, expressive or receptive dysphasia.

INVESTIGATIONS

Diagnostic investigations may include:

- MRI scan (magnetic resonance imaging)
- CT scan (computed tomography)
- neurological examination
- PET scan (positron emission tomography)
- brain angiogram
- EEG (electroencephalogram)
- biopsy.

MEDICAL TREATMENTS

- Surgery – If the tumour can be removed without undue risk of neurological damage and subsequent functional implications, surgical intervention such as a craniotomy will be performed to achieve resection or partial debulking.
- Radiotherapy – The dose and number of fractions administered differ for primary and metastatic tumours. Radiotherapy is given to increase the chance of disease control, prevent recurrence or for palliative purposes. This can be administered as radical radiotherapy or as a palliative (hypo-fractionated) dose.
- Chemotherapy – The role of chemotherapy continues to be investigated through drug trials, which currently concentrate on primary astrocytic tumours. The brain is unique in that it is protected by the blood–brain barrier and therefore there are limited chemotherapy treatments that can permeate these membranes. Chemotherapy can be a single or combined agent and is often used for recurring gliomas.
- Steroids – Drugs such as dexamethasone are used to reduce intracranial pressure caused by cerebral oedema or inflammation around the spinal cord. These are often a time-limited treatment due to the high risk of adverse side-effects.

Anti-convulsant and anti-emetic medications are used to prevent seizures and to alleviate nausea.

SIDE-EFFECTS OF TREATMENTS

The treatments used in the management of CNS tumours can cause side-effects that consequently affect function, for example:

- surgery – post-operation fatigue, inflammation around surgical site causing numerous temporary deficits and/or long-term residual damage;
- radiotherapy – fatigue, somnolence, alopecia;
- chemotherapy – fatigue, nausea and vomiting;
- steroids – water retention, proximal myopathy, cushingoid appearance, fragile skin, steroid-induced diabetes.

OCCUPATIONAL THERAPY ASSESSMENT

For clients with CNS tumours, participation in self-care, productivity and leisure may be affected by physical, cognitive and psychological impairment that in turn impacts on roles and social activities. Clients present to rehabilitation services with a spectrum of deficits. These can prove to be some of the most challenging cancer diagnoses for professionals (Kirshblum *et al.*, 2001). Comprehensive assessment of the client as a whole will focus on a number of distinct but interlinking aspects of function.

PHYSICAL ASSESSMENT

Physical assessment should investigate the effect of altered muscle strength, joint range of movement, muscle tone, balance, coordination, sensation, proprioception and pain on function. If possible, an initial physical assessment together with a physiotherapist enables a comprehensive assessment while also limiting the unnecessary repetition of information and preventing the client from becoming exhausted. It will be important to establish how much active movement the client is able to achieve, as well as assessing passive range of movement and identifying any impeding factors such as contractures or high/low tone. Depending on the area of the brain or spinal cord affected, clients may also present with hemiplegia, unsteady gait, tremor, and focal or global weakness. As stated, some treatment modalities, such as steroids, can cause physical changes such as a cushingoid appearance and proximal myopathies. Visual disturbances may also occur, e.g. diplopia or hemianopia.

The occupational therapist must be aware of the client's trunk stability, as this will influence which activities are to be chosen when planning treatment. It is also useful to know about the client's previous level of functioning and any premorbid conditions that may influence participation in activities. A comprehensive assessment is carried out by observing the client engaging in activities from their daily routine, such as dressing, transferring on/off their chair, reading the newspaper or pouring a glass of water from a jug. Such activities will help identify any problems with muscle strength, coordination, balance and sensation and may be more purposeful for the client than simply assessing movement in isolation.

Fatigue is likely to be a major factor for the client and it is advisable to be aware of its impact on their daily routine. Ascertaining if there is any pattern to the fatigue and which times of the day are best for the client will assist in successful planning of treatment as well as incorporating fatigue management strategies. Somnolence describes the extreme exhaustion that patients can experience as a result of radiotherapy. This debilitating symptom may emerge after the treatment and can last for six to eight weeks after the completion of radiotherapy (Guerrero, 1998). The severity of the somnolence can make it very difficult for patients to undertake activities of daily living effectively and to attend hospital appointments. Talking to clients and their families before, during and after radiotherapy treatment is important to forewarn them and support them through a symptom that can render the individual physically and emotionally low.

COGNITIVE ASSESSMENT

Cognition refers to the mental processes that enable individuals to make sense of the world around them. In assessment the therapist should consider the following hierarchy of cognitive skills (Malia and Brannagan, 2000):

- Attention – Underpinning all other cognitive processes, this describes the ability to focus, shift and divide attention between different tasks. Problems may include being easily distracted, inability to concentrate for an extended period of time or on more than one thing, losing track in the middle of a task or conversation.
- Visual processing – This involves seeing and the interpretation of this information. Problems may include spatial awareness, lack of clarity, limitation of the field of vision and inability to match new visual information with that previously stored.
- Memory – This is a process that involves retaining information and recalling this at a later stage. Problems may include forgetting information (e.g. names, conversation topics, appointment times, personal history) or remembering how to complete tasks.
- Information processing – This could be defined as the assimilation of sensory and other information to interpret the environment. Problems may include a delay in responding, keeping up with conversations, and confusion in busy situations.
- Executive functions – Skills such as problem solving, goal setting, initiation, planning and organization come under this category and are considered to be the higher-level cognitive functions. Problems may include difficulties with insight, monitoring behaviour and self-awareness.

Problems as identified above may also have an impact on behaviour, which in turn can affect the emotional welfare of the client and those around them. Sherwood *et al.* (2004) highlighted the strain on family members caring for an individual with a brain tumour. Their study found that for carers, trying to manage cognitive and neuropsychiatric sequelae was the most difficult aspect of caring.

PSYCHOLOGICAL AND SOCIAL ASSESSMENT

The brain is the organ that 'more than any other is linked to our sense of self' (Kibler, 1998) and the diagnosis of a brain tumour, subsequent effects of disease and treatment can have a devastating impact on psychological well-being. The shock of a life-threatening diagnosis and possible physical, cognitive, behavioural and personality changes can place pressure on the family and carers. Roles within a family or social network may be significantly altered (Bauscwein *et al.*, 2004). Communication problems may hamper interaction and the inability to articulate needs may lead to frustration. Furthermore, effects of treatment such as hair loss or substantial weight change can lead to anxieties about an altered body image.

The diagnosis of a life-limiting condition heralds anxiety and fear for the client and family. This anxiety can be exacerbated by the numerous appointments to be attended, waiting for scan results, and planning for treatment involving procedures such as the moulding masks for radiotherapy. An aggressive tumour can denote a severely limited prognosis. Those with a low-grade tumour may live with a more protracted wait and threat of disease progression. Support for the client and family is essential in facilitating the adjustment to multiple losses throughout the phases of the disease trajectory and coming to terms with the prospect of a limited prognosis.

RANGE OF ASSESSMENTS

A number of standardized assessments are available for use with clients in this setting such as the Canadian Occupational Performance Measure (COPM) (Law et al., 2005); the Assessment of Motor and Processing Skills (Fisher, 2001a and b); the Cognitive Assessment of Minnesota (Rustad et al., 1993); the Chessington Occupational Therapy Neurological Assessment Battery (Tyerman et al., 1986); and the Rivermead Assessments (Whiting and Lincoln, 1980). No one tool can provide the definitive assessment and it may be necessary to carry out a range of assessments. However, it is important to be sensitive to the particular needs of the client, and the occupational therapist must consider any limiting effects, e.g. fatigue. Though it is promoted that assessments should be carried out in full it will often be necessary to use separate elements of a lengthy assessment, recognizing this compromises validity and reliability. Before carrying out any assessment the occupational therapist must be clear as to the rationale for using it and the benefit this will have for the client.

Observing clients participating in a purposeful activity will provide a thorough assessment of their function. Safety concerns may be highlighted when carrying out activities of daily living such as managing medications and undertaking tasks in the kitchen. Assessment of the home environment will provide the opportunity to minimize risk and consider aids and adaptations. Another method is to use questionnaires that can be given to the client or carer to establish a premorbid level of functioning and current abilities and concerns.

Bye (1998) recognizes that occupational therapists may reframe their approach to assessment for clients with a life-limiting condition. Assessment can be kept low-key so that a client is not pushed to perform in all activities of daily living to examine functioning. Indeed, as function declines the occupational therapist may alter the emphasis of assessment to focus on the carer's ability to manage and support the client. For professionals to address the complex needs of clients with brain tumours, it is important that occupational therapists adopt a client-centred approach and work as a team on common goals.

OCCUPATIONAL THERAPY INTERVENTION

When planning a treatment programme, clear rehabilitation goals should be set by the client and occupational therapist, involving family members and other professionals as appropriate. Having identified goals with the client, a treatment programme may involve working on maximizing independence in personal care, domestic tasks, productivity and leisure activities or providing the individual with effective coping strategies to manage problems such as fatigue, cognitive deficits or reduced self-confidence.

Many of the principles of neuro-rehabilitation that can be applied to individuals with stroke, traumatic brain or spinal cord injury can be applied to those with brain and CNS tumours (Kirshblum et al., 2001). However, rehabilitation programmes need to be tailored to the specific needs of clients with neurological cancers, accommodating chemotherapy and radiotherapy treatments and their effects, particularly fatigue (Bell et al., 1998).

Rehabilitation can take place in an inpatient or outpatient setting or in the client's home (National Council for Hospice and Specialist Palliative Care Services, 2000). Beck (2003) recognized that admission to rehabilitation units should depend on an individual's life goals within the context of their prognosis. Rehabilitation in neuro-oncology provides a challenge for the occupational therapist as the client may have a limited prognosis and any time spent in therapy will need to be balanced with the time the client chooses to spend otherwise.

Time frames for intervention can be shorter than for the rehabilitation of individuals with different diagnoses (Kirshblum et al., 2001). Garrard et al. (2004) extol the collaboration of rehabilitation and palliative care services and their shared ethos that focuses on alleviating symptoms, enhancing independence and quality of life. Evidence that focuses on inpatient admissions suggests that patients with brain tumours do benefit from rehabilitative intervention (Huang et al., 2000; Kirshblum et al., 2001; Marciniak et al., 2001; Garrard et al., 2004).

PHYSICAL INTERVENTION

An individual with a CNS tumour can present with many physical manifestations as a result of the damage to the brain or spinal cord. The occupational therapist's focus is to optimize function while assessing safety in a client population that can have reduced insight and problem-solving capacities. For these clients presenting with hemiplegia and such impairments, it is, as ever, important to use meaningful activities for treatment, e.g. using washing, dressing or food preparation to facilitate normal movement, encourage use of weaker limbs or increase awareness of a neglected side. Purposeful tasks aim to build up or maintain activity tolerance and muscle strength. Specific graded activities can focus on maintenance or return of function in upper limbs. These may develop from tasks undertaken in sitting, progressing to standing.

Where problems are evident, it is important to establish safe methods of transferring and mobility in conjunction with the physiotherapist. It is vital to involve family and carers in any training regarding safe manual handling techniques and the use of any assistive equipment such as sliding sheets and hoists. If mobility is severely compromised, it may be necessary to carry out a posture and seating assessment in order to provide an appropriate wheelchair and pressure-relieving cushions.

Sometimes it may be necessary to provide equipment to assist with activities of daily living and minimize any risk, e.g. bathing equipment. Smaller aids will often be helpful in maintaining independence with activities such as writing, eating and cooking, e.g. pen grips, large-grip cutlery (for those with upper limb weakness) or liquid level indicators (for those with visual deficits).

Advice on managing fatigue is often helpful and principles of energy conservation, balancing activity and rest and adapting activities as discussed in the chapter on fatigue management, can be taught. Giving written information and working with carers may be useful when working with clients who have compromised cognitive skills.

COGNITIVE INTERVENTION

Although numerous tools and strategies exist for cognitive rehabilitation, the challenges encountered with this particular client group mean that the emphasis for the occupational therapist will often be on maintaining functional activities, devising compensatory strategies and ensuring safety through risk assessment. Education of the client and carer is vital in engaging them in a therapeutic programme that is effective.

Minimizing distractions by removing background noise (television, radio, conversation) and limiting interruptions can help with attention and concentration. The client may become overwhelmed and overloaded with lots of information. Avoiding complex instructions can help maintain attention and facilitate information processing. Use of diaries, lists, electronic alarms or aids may help to compensate for memory loss, for example using a watch alarm to prompt with medication. Having written instructions around the home for certain tasks such as using the washing machine may encourage clients to maintain activities important to their role and routine.

To focus the client's attention, the occupational therapist can use verbal prompts, for example 'I remember you said before . . .' or 'before going on to do that . . .'. The occupational therapist should not be afraid to interrupt or move back to the main point, for example, 'yes, shall we come back to that?'. As well as external prompts the client can also employ internal strategies such as self-questioning ('what should I be doing now?') or mental rehearsal of planned tasks.

Perceptual problems, such as apraxia or inattention, may also be addressed by a compensatory approach. Educating clients and carers and increasing awareness when there are problems will assist in the management of such deficits. For example, if a client has a left-sided inattention, strategies may involve verbal prompts to ensure that they do not walk into objects on their left side, encouraging scanning with their head to ensure that things on the left side are seen, or using written reminders for safety, e.g. checking the temperature of bath water before getting in.

As clients' safety can be compromised by lack of insight or other deficits, it is important for the occupational therapist to assess their ability to function safely at home, e.g. in the kitchen, administration of medication, their risk of falling and orientation outside the home.

PSYCHOLOGICAL AND SOCIAL INTERVENTION

An important starting point is to offer support and education for the client and family regarding their diagnosis, side-effects and functional implications, which can help in alleviating confusion and misunderstanding. Listening to the client and carer and offering advice and interventions when they are ready to receive it can help with the establishment of a good therapeutic relationship. Clients with high-grade diagnoses face the consequence of aggressive disease. For others with low-grade diagnoses, the prospect of living with a more prolonged but still life-limiting condition can bring with it particular stresses. For this client group, often young adults, they may be dealing with seizures, taking medications, attending hospital appointments, as well as coping with changes in body image or personality. These factors can affect their family, social and working lives leading to relationship, psychological or financial worries while living with the anxiety about progressive disease.

The loss of function and roles for a client, as well as loss of health and years, will mean that occupational therapists are often present when they experience difficulty in undertaking previously straightforward tasks. This means that they must be prepared to help someone adjust to functional deterioration within the context of multiple losses. Professionals may observe a range of emotions from individuals (frustration, anger, depression, fear, etc.) and the consequent impact on relationships. Occupational therapists can offer relaxation training and anxiety management to patients who may experience anxiety and distress in stressful circumstances. Referral on to other team members, e.g. clinical psychologists or counsellors, may also be appropriate.

EVALUATION OF INTERVENTION

Evaluation of occupational therapy intervention should tie in with methods of assessment. Reassessment with a standardized tool will provide an outcome measure to evaluate the interventions. As it is not always appropriate to carry out such measures, the occupational therapist must ensure that the agreed goals are realistic and reflect the client's changing priorities. It will be natural to see a fluctuating and deteriorating picture of function of which the client can be acutely aware. If using an assessment that incorporates a satisfaction score, such as the COPM, this may reflect the client's increased ability to cope with the situation rather than that any functional improvements have been made.

CASE STUDIES

CASE STUDY 1

Mr A

Age at onset: 45

Diagnosis: Left frontal parietal glioblastoma multiforme grade IV

Past medical history: Mr A first presented to his GP with a history of headaches, nausea and vomiting. Other symptoms experienced were focal seizures, lack of coordination, bumping into things on the right-hand side, short-term memory loss and expressive dysphasia. Mr A had a craniotomy and debulking of tumour, followed by 30 fractions of radical radiotherapy and two cycles of chemotherapy. The headaches, nausea and vomiting initially ceased, seizures were controlled by anti-convulsant medication and coordination problems and dysphasia resolved.

Social history: Mr A lived with his wife and had two adult children. A commercial driver by profession, the diagnosis had resulted in him having to give up work; Mr A was receiving appropriate benefits.

OCCUPATIONAL THERAPY INTERVENTION:

First referral to the hospital occupational therapist was received upon completion of radiotherapy as Mr A was experiencing anxiety and panic attacks.

Initial assessment revealed that Mr A was very motivated to learn strategies to manage his anxiety and panic attacks. His anxiety was impacting on his function to the extent that he no longer felt able to go outside alone due to the risk of fits. Mr A participated in a six-session programme of anxiety management which included identifying triggers of anxiety, recognizing 'normal' reactions to his current situation, challenging negative thoughts in a constructive way and teaching relaxation techniques. Agreed goals were set with Mr A practising relaxation techniques and strategies learned in the sessions. After the initial six sessions and a follow-up session a month later, Mr A felt confident enough to employ anxiety management strategies, was feeling confident enough to go out for short periods unaccompanied and was discharged from occupational therapy.

Six months later, Mr A began to experience symptoms of right-sided weakness and recurrence of his dysphasia. Following investigations, he was given two further cycles of chemotherapy, which were abandoned due to further disease progression. Mr A was then admitted to a local oncology unit for further investigations and rehabilitation.

Assessment proved challenging as Mr A was dysphasic but Mrs A was involved. The process was aided by the fact that the occupational therapist had previously built up a therapeutic relationship with Mr A. Goals for therapy intervention were agreed with Mr A, the occupational therapist, physiotherapist and speech and language therapist. His priorities were to be able to go to the toilet independently and to be able to return home. Mr A required assistance in walking due to his right-sided weakness and his safety in transfers was also compromised by his impaired awareness of safety and lack of insight into his current difficulties. The occupational therapist worked on a consistent approach to safe transfers, then progressed to independent transfers. An attendant-propelled (9L) wheelchair was provided to enable Mr A to get to the toilet safely, where he could be left to transfer on to the toilet independently and manage his own personal hygiene. The physiotherapist continued to work on walking, providing Mr A with an ankle foot orthosis.

A home assessment was carried out with Mr and Mrs A and risks identified. Assistive equipment such as a wheeled commode, toilet frame, bath lift and chair raisers were provided and advice given regarding management around the home. Mr A was at risk of falls and required supervision for safety but both Mr and Mrs A were determined for him to return home realizing that his prognosis, by this stage, was poor.

After one month at home, Mr A's condition progressed further, resulting in the need to be admitted to the oncology unit again, this time for terminal care. Mr A died 13 days later, comfortably and in the presence of his family.

CASE STUDY 2

Mrs B

Age at onset: 39

Diagnosis: Breast cancer with cerebral metastases

Past medical history: Diagnosed with breast cancer and underwent a lumpectomy, chemotherapy and radiotherapy. Two years later cerebral metastases were diagnosed following symptoms of right-sided weakness and dysphasia. Mrs B was started on steroids and underwent whole brain radiotherapy. Since then she has been maintained on steroids and anti-convulsion medication.

Social history: Mrs B lives with her husband and two teenage children. She worked as a secretary. Her parents live nearby and are supportive.

OCCUPATIONAL THERAPY INTERVENTION:

First referral to the hospice occupational therapist was received following radiotherapy for the cerebral metastases. Mrs B was experiencing problems with mobilizing and transferring safely around her home due to reduced power, coordination and proprioception in her right arm and leg.

An initial assessment was carried out at home. Mrs B was mobile with a walking stick and still working at this stage. The main problems she identified were fatigue, getting into/out of the bath safely, managing the stairs and outside step and using her right arm. Following assessment, Mrs B was provided with a bath lift. Stair rails were installed and advice given on safe negotiation on the stairs, which Mrs B was still managing independently. A half step was put in place at the front door. The occupational therapist recommended activities to encourage movement of the right arm and advice was given on the management of high tone that was present.

Advice was given on managing fatigue, specifically in relation to continuing working and reduced hours. Small work-related goals were agreed. Mrs B stated that it was important for her to remain at work for as long as possible even if this meant just visiting work to meet with colleagues as this enabled her to maintain her sense of self. Mrs B's employers were very supportive in helping her with this plan. Mr and Mrs B were having a downstairs toilet and shower room installed and advice was also given on the type of flooring, height of toilet and positioning of rails. After two follow-up visits, Mrs B was discharged from occupational therapy.

One month later, Mrs B was re-referred to the occupational therapist as she was experiencing further problems with managing personal
hygiene, outdoor mobility and had fallen at home. A home visit was
carried out and Mrs B tried using a shower chair in the downstairs
shower room which proved easier than using the bath. A raised toilet
seat was provided for the toilet and further rails were installed upstairs
and in the bathroom. Mrs B was struggling with managing the stairs but
was keen to continue sleeping upstairs as she felt this retained a sense
of normality for her and her family. The occupational therapist advised
Mr B on how to supervise Mrs B safely when negotiating the stairs. Mrs
B agreed to provision of a wheelchair for outdoor use and was referred
to the local wheelchair service. The occupational therapist also referred
Mrs B to the physiotherapist for assessment for a different walking aid
as she was having difficulty walking with a stick. Mrs B was by this stage
attending a hospice day centre, which enabled the occupational therapist
to keep in regular contact to monitor the situation. Two months later,
Mrs B reported having difficulties with bed transfers and feeding. The
occupational therapist assessed Mrs B with adapted cutlery and provided her with a set to try at home. She was also provided with a bed
lever to assist with bed transfers. Mrs B had stopped working by this
stage. The occupational therapist went through fatigue management
principles for home and gave advice on pacing and prioritizing
activities.

After another month, Mrs B was admitted to a hospice inpatient
unit for rehabilitation as things were becoming increasingly difficult at
home. This admission was also an opportunity to explore whether Mr
and Mrs B would like to have any formal care on discharge, something
they had previously declined. The occupational therapist was involved
again in setting up the environment on the unit to try to make it as much
like home as possible, ensuring the bed lever and any other relevant
equipment was available and fitted. Rehabilitation goals were set with
Mrs B, the occupational therapist, the physiotherapist, the speech and
language therapist and the nursing team. Mrs B was at risk of falls and
needed supervision to walk using her tripod frame but was still insistent
on remaining as independent as possible, including walking up and
down the stairs. Intervention involved practising transfers and activities,
which ensured safety while also maintaining a level of independence.
Mrs B was discharged home after nine days. The occupational therapist
carried out a follow-up visit and adjustments were made to the home
such as placing commodes next to the bed and chair and providing a
riser recliner armchair to assist with transfers and positioning during
the day.

It has been important through the time that the occupational therapist has been involved with Mrs B to enable her to identify her own problems and agree common goals. It has also been important to introduce the concept of equipment gradually to encourage acceptance and to support Mrs B's wish to be as independent as possible. Mrs B is still attending the day centre and regularly monitored by the occupational therapist.

SUMMARY

Occupational therapy has a clear role in the treatment of CNS tumours, both in the acute and palliative stages. However, this client group raises a real challenge to the occupational therapist as many complex factors can impact upon rehabilitation. Although techniques used in other areas of neuro-rehabilitation can be effectively employed, the occupational therapist must be aware of the unique issues that are relevant to this particular client group. The client's performance may vary according to the stage of disease or treatment regime they are undergoing. Limiting factors such as fatigue or cognitive problems may compromise effective intervention. Involvement with this client population also requires sensitivity to the psychological and emotional issues that individuals and their families may be experiencing, bearing in mind the adjustments that need to be made in an often limited period of time. The aims and objectives of intervention should be sufficiently flexible to enable the occupational therapist to work with the client and family at any stage of their disease trajectory.

ACTION POINTS

1. A patient with a brain tumour is referred for relaxation but has memory difficulties. What approach would the occupational therapist take in developing an anxiety management and relaxation programme in which family members or carers would be involved?
2. A female patient with a young family has radiotherapy-induced somnolence; this is causing functional difficulties for her at home, and also adding strain to the family dynamics. What advice would the occupational therapist give to the family to be able to adapt and cope with this fatigue?
3. Consider particular elements of occupational therapy assessments and discuss which are relevant for patients with brain tumours with short attention spans and difficulty concentrating.

REFERENCES

Bausewein, C., Borasio, G. D. and Voltz, R. (2004) Brain tumours. *Oxford Textbook of Palliative Medicine*, 3rd edn (eds D. Doyle, G. Hanks, N. Cherry and K. Calman), Oxford University Press, Oxford.

Beck, L. A. (2003) Cancer rehabilitation: Does it make a difference? *Rehabilitation Nursing*, **28**(2), 42–7.

Bell, K. R., O'Dell, M. W., Barr, K. and Yablon, S. A. (1998) Rehabilitation of the patient with brain tumor. *Archives of Physical Medicine and Rehabilitation*, **3**(Suppl 1), 37–48.

Bye, R. A. (1998) When clients are dying: Occupational therapists' perspectives. *The Occupational Therapy Journal of Research*, **18**(1), 3–24.

Cancer Research UK (2005) accessed July 2005 on www.cancerresearchuk.org

Fisher, A. G. (2001a) *Assessment of Motor and Process Skills (AMPS): Development, standardization, and administration manual*, 4th edn, vol. **1**, Three Star Press, London.

Fisher, A. G. (2001b) *Assessment of Motor and Process Skills (AMPS): User manual*, 4th edn, vol. **2**, Three Star Press, London.

Garrard, P., Farnham, C., Thompson, A. J. and Playford, E. D. (2004) Rehabilitation of the cancer patient: Experience in a neurological unit. *Neuro-rehabilitation and Neuro Repair*, **18**(2), 76–9.

Guerrero, D. (1998) *Neuro-Oncology for Nurses*, Whurr, London.

Hill, C. I., Nixon, C. S., Ruehmeier, J. L. and Wolf, L. M. (2002) Brain tumors. *Physical Therapy*, **82**(5), 496–502.

Huang, M. E., Cifu, D. X. and Keyser-Marcus, L. (2000) Functional outcomes in patients with brain tumor after inpatient rehabilitation: Comparison with traumatic brain injury. *American Journal of Physical Medicine and Rehabilitation*, **79**(4), 327–35.

Kibler, S. (1998) Psychological support. *Neuro-oncology for Nurses* (ed. D. Guerro), Whurr, London.

Kirshblum, S., O'Dell, M. W., Ho, C. and Barr, K. (2001) Rehabilitation of persons with central nervous system tumors. *Cancer*, **92**(S4), 1029–38.

Kleihues, P., Burger, P. C. and Scheithauer, B. W. (1993) The new WHO classification of brain tumours. *Brain Pathology*, **3**(3), 255–68.

Law, M., Baptiste, S., Carswell, A., McColl, M. A., Polatajko, H. and Pollock, N. (2005) *Canadian Occupational Performance Measure*, Canadian Association of Occupational Therapists, Ontario.

Malia, K. and Brannagan, A. (2000) *Cognitive Rehabilitation Workshop for Professionals*, Braintree, Epsom.

Marciniak, C. M., Silwa, J. A., Heinemann, A. W. and Semik, P. E. (2001) Functional outcomes of persons with brain tumors after inpatient rehabilitation. *Archives of Physical Medicine and Rehabilitation*, **82**(4), 457–63.

National Council for Hospice and Specialist Palliative Care Services (2000) *Fulfilling Lives: Rehabilitation in palliative care*, Land & Unwin Ltd, Northamptonshire.

Rustad, R. A., DeGroot, T. L., Jungkunz, M. L., Freeberg, K. S., Borowick, L. G. and Wanttie, A. M. (1993) *The Cognitive Assessment of Minnesota*, Therapy Skill Builders, Texas.

Sherwood, P. R., Given, B. A., Doorenbos, A. Z. and Given, G. W. (2004) Forgotten voices: Lessons from bereaved caregivers of persons with a brain tumour. *International Journal of Palliative Nursing*, **10**(2), 67–75.

Soo, E. W., Galindo, E. G. and Levin, V. A. (1997) A comprehensive review of brain tumours: www.cancernetwork.com/textbook/morev30.htm

Tyerman, R., Tyerman, A., Howard, P. and Hadfield, C. (1986) *Chessington OT Neurological Assessment Battery (COTNAB)*, Nottingham Rehab, Nottingham.

Wen, P. Y. and Loeffler, J. S. (1999) Management of brain metastases. *Oncology*, **13**(7), 941–54, 957–61.

Whiting, S. and Lincoln, N. (1980) Rivermead activities of daily living (RADL): An ADL assessment for stroke patients. *British Journal of Occupational Therapy*, **43**(1), 44–6.

RECOMMENDED READING

Cooper, J. (1997) *Occupational Therapy in Oncology and Palliative Care*, Whurr, London.

Huang, M. E., Wartella, J. E. and Kreutzer, J. S. (2001) Functional outcomes and quality of life in patients with brain tumors: A preliminary report. *Archives of Physical Medicine and Rehabilitation*, **82**(11), 1540–6.

Mukand, J. A., Guilmette, T. J. and Tran, M. (2003) Rehabilitation for patients with brain tumors. *Critical Reviews in Physical and Rehabilitation Medicine*, **15**(2), 99–111.

Whiting, S., Lincoln, N., Bhavani, G. and Cockburn, J. (1985) *Rivermead Perceptual Assessment Battery (RPAB)*, NFER-Nelson, Windsor.

Wilson, B., Cockburn, J. and Baddeley, A. (1991) *The Rivermead Behavioural Memory Test (RBMT)*, Thames Valley Test Company, Bury St Edmunds.

11 Occupational Therapy in Hospices and Day Care

ANNE BOSTOCK, SHELLEY ELLIS, SARA MATHEWSON
AND LILIAS METHVEN

Bray (1997) describes how, historically, health care has followed a biomedical model, focusing on disease and the physical symptoms of disease. Hospice care has followed a more client-centred approach, focusing on the bio–psycho-social, and latterly spiritual aspects of care.

Hospices can be traced to medieval times when, it is suggested, they were established along pilgrim routes where they welcomed travellers, pilgrims, orphans and the destitute, as well as the sick and dying. Doctors did not associate themselves with such institutions as it was thought unethical to treat a patient with a 'deadly' disease. After all, they had their reputations to consider. The word 'hospice' was first used to describe the care given to the dying by Mme Jeanne Garnier in Lyons, France, in 1842. The Irish Sisters of Charity established Our Lady's Hospice in 1879 and later St Joseph's Hospice in East London in 1905. At about the same time other religious centres established care for the sick and dying throughout the country in what were commonly known as 'homes for the dying'.

The Marie Curie Memorial Foundation was established in 1948 and aimed to provide care for cancer patients dying at home with support from Marie Curie community nurses. Later a series of homes, which are now recognized as palliative care centres, were opened by the Foundation.

Developments in the hospice movement in the 1950s coincided with other medical developments: the discovery of new psychotrophic drugs, the phenothiazines, antidepressants and the anxiolytics, as well as the development of synthetic steroid and non-steroidal anti-inflammatory drugs, and developments in chemotherapy and intensive care units.

The philosophy of hospice and palliative care demonstrates a generalist approach to the patient and family that is different from the specialist approach of the medical model of health care (Dawson and Barker, 1995). The principles of hospice care have extended out of the physical hospice building into the community and also into the acute setting. Care is directed towards maintaining quality of life for the patient and family, so enabling the patient to

Occupational Therapy in Oncology and Palliative Care. Edited by J. Cooper
© 2006 John Wiley & Sons Ltd

remain at home. Recent trends in literature about palliative care describe the value of hospice care:

> ... helps the patient and their family to cope with disease progression and treatment of it – from pre-diagnosis, through the process of diagnosis and treatment, to cure, continuing illness or death and into bereavement. It helps the patient to maximize the benefits of treatment and to live as well as possible with the effects of the disease. It is given equal priority alongside treatment and diagnosis.
>
> (NCHSPCS, 2002)

Palliative care has long been associated with the hospice movement; however, it too has continued to develop and was recognized in 1987 as a specialty of medicine in Great Britain. The World Health Organization (2002) defines palliative care as:

> ... an approach that improves the quality of life of patients and their families facing the problem associated with life-threatening illness, through the prevention and relief of suffering by means of early identification and impeccable as–sessment and treatment of pain and other problems, physical, psychosocial and spiritual ... Palliative care provides relief from pain and other distressing symptoms; affirms life and regards dying as a normal process, integrates the psychological and spiritual aspects of patient care; offers a support system to help the family cope during the patient's illness and in their own bereavement; uses a team approach to address the needs of the patient and their families.
>
> (WHO, 2002)

Traditionally, hospices and palliative care have been associated with the needs of cancer patients and families. However, this now extends to those with any progressive illness, as patients will undoubtedly benefit from the principles and management of palliative care. This applies to conditions such as multiple sclerosis, motor neurone disease, muscular dystrophy and other neurological conditions, chronic heart failure, and in more recent years the challenge of HIV/AIDS.

Hospices or palliative care units in Britain are funded by the National Health Service, or large national or local charities receiving some assistance from the National Health Service. Currently there are 172 specialist in-patient units in England, of which 130 are funded by the voluntary sector and 42 are managed by the National Health Service (House of Commons, 2004, p. 4). Hospices vary in size, structure and service provision. Services range from inpatient care, day care, outpatient clinics (medical consultation, lymphoedema management), domiciliary support from any member of the multidisciplinary team and specialist nurse advisors (home care teams) and hospice-at-home teams. Centres offer some or all of these services. Care is provided by an extensive multidisciplinary team including doctors, nurses, social workers, physiotherapists, occupational therapists, chaplains, bereavement workers and volunteers. Occupational therapy complements the skill mix of the multidisciplinary team.

The philosophy of the profession encompasses the principles of palliative care as defined by the World Health Organization (2002). Although the recognition and employment of occupational therapists throughout hospices and palliative care units continues to grow, it is still subject to local variation.

The National Council for Hospice and Specialist Palliative Care Services (1995) Statement of Definitions advises that specialist services should have a state registered occupational therapist available full time, part time or with regular sessions. This should encourage existing and developing palliative care services to incorporate occupational therapy into their multiprofessional team (Department of Health, 2000; National Council for Hospice and Specialist Palliative Care Services, 2002).

OCCUPATIONAL THERAPY MODEL

The Human Occupations model (Reed and Sanderson, 1988) identifies the individual as the central element in occupational therapy intervention. The occupational therapist identifies the unique processes, concepts, techniques, concerns and assumptions and ultimately the outcomes of occupational therapy. The focus is on 'wellness' but this is not based on a medical model. The assessment addresses the individual's occupations, which are defined as meaning any activity requiring the individual's time and energy and thus using skills that have a value (a learned behaviour or a belief in something, for example). These occupations are related to self-maintenance, productivity and leisure. The individual must be able to participate in assessment and treatment and must also have the necessary components to carry out these occupations, these components being motor, sensory, cognitive, intrapersonal and interpersonal. These are defined as:

- motor skills – the level, quality and/or degree of range of motion, gross muscle strength, muscle tone, endurance, fine motor skills and functional use of these;
- sensory skills – concerned with perceiving and differentiating external and internal stimuli;
- cognitive skills – the level, quality and/or degree of comprehension, communication, concentration, problem solving, time management, conceptualization, integration of learning, judgement and time/place/person orientation;
- intrapersonal skills – the level, quality and/or degree of self-identity, self-concept and coping;
- interpersonal skills – the level, quality and/or degree of dyadic and group interaction.

The next level of skills are:

- self-maintenance occupations – those activities or tasks that are carried out routinely to maintain the client's health and well-being in the environment, such as dressing or eating;
- productivity occupations – those activities or tasks that are carried out to enable clients to provide support to themselves, their families and society;
- leisure occupations – those activities or tasks carried out for the enjoyment and renewal that the activity or task brings to the client. They may contribute to the promotion of health and well-being (Townsend *et al.*, 1997; Lyons *et al.*, 2002).

MOTOR SKILLS

For many patients these skills are affected by muscle wastage or weakness which may be due to weight loss or weight gain. The result of this on the patient is loss of range of movement, a reduction in the ease of transfers or general mobility and fatigue. The early introduction and supply of equipment (for example, toileting aids) may benefit a person's independence, thus giving them a positive experience (Soderback and Paulsson, 1997). As patients decline they may require additional support from a carer or professional. If equipment is supplied in the latter stages of decline, this can be viewed negatively by an individual and reinforce the progress of their disease.

This also applies to the use and supply of wheelchairs. Individuals may benefit from the supply of a wheelchair for long-distance outdoor use when they have reduced energy levels and fatigue, however mobile they may be around their own homes and garden. Positive experiences and pleasurable memories all ease acceptance when the patient is limited further.

General advice can be given by the occupational therapist on energy conservation, how activities can be spread throughout the day, limiting stair climbing, and sitting while carrying out activities. Alternative techniques for carrying out activities can also be taught.

It is important to establish the patients' priorities, getting them to set the goals, to focus on the important activities, and to accept help from others in completing the less-important tasks.

SENSORY SKILLS

Patients experience many different degrees and varieties of pain and often a patient's pain can be described as 'total pain', the focus of which may not be a physical sensation. It is important to recognize the width of the concept of pain and its influence over the occupations and activity when implementing occupational therapy assessment and treatment programmes. This may mean coordinating the timing of the treatment sessions prior to administering medication to facilitate optimal functioning.

Patients may have distorted sensation or a loss of sensation as a result of tumour growth on a nerve, or fibrosing of tissue, or they may have a medically induced loss of sensation for pain control. For these patients, advice and supply of equipment may be necessary to prevent accidental damage, for example when undertaking kitchen activities.

Loss of sensation decreases the patient's awareness of the development of pressure sores (the pain from such sores can have a dramatic effect on a person's well-being). The supply of appropriate cushions and mattresses is essential to the prevention of pressure sores. Occupational therapists have a wealth of knowledge on a wide range of pressure-relieving cushions.

COGNITIVE SKILLS

Cognitive impairment may be a direct result of tumour growth within the brain or secondary growths. It may be as a result of side-effects from medication or dramatic effects of fatigue. Those with direct tumour growth require a sound occupational therapy neurological assessment prior to implementing a treatment programme.

All aspects of communication, comprehension, concentration and organizational skills need to be assessed by the occupational therapist as these are vital to the performance of occupations. For example, preparing a meal requires organization, concentration, ability to sequence task and problem-solving skills. Perceptual skills also play an important role in this task, e.g. ability to judge objects on a kitchen worktop and putting food into a saucepan.

INTRAPERSONAL SKILLS

Poor self-image can inhibit drastically an individual's ability to cope with the 'occupations' and activities required in life. Feelings of anxiety and stress should be recognized and relaxation programmes should be taught to develop coping mechanisms to deal with such feelings in everyday life.

Patients whose occupational performance is affected by their intrapersonal skills may need additional psychological support from specialized clinicians, e.g. a psychologist. In such situations the occupational therapist should refer the client to appropriate agencies. Goal setting has the positive benefit of facilitating patients' involvement in, and subsequent control of, their lives (MacLaren, 1996).

INTERPERSONAL SKILLS

The disease often becomes the focus of patients' lives. They become disease-orientated, they lose control of their lives, they lose their roles, and in turn they lose self-confidence, self-worth and self-respect (Vrkljan and Miller-Polgar, 2001). This is why patients should be encouraged to set goals – it gives them some control over their lives and increases their motivation and their positive feelings of self-worth. The use of a structured programme of activity within hospice day care can use group work constructively to enhance these positive feelings. Having addressed the performance components or skills required by the individual, one then focuses on the occupational components, the activities in routine daily life.

SELF-MAINTENANCE

This includes the skills necessary for personal activities of daily living: washing, bathing, dressing and toileting; and domestic activities: shopping, cooking, laundry, cleaning and general household duties. The occupational therapist might assess with the patient issues with self-maintenance tasks if this is identified by the individual as a personal goal. These goals should then be addressed by the occupational therapist as to how the patient will achieve them (Wilcock *et al.*, 1997). The occupational therapist can correct underlying problems, teach alternative methods or supply equipment in order to maintain independence. Those activities that are not deemed to be a priority to the patient could be carried out by a carer or professional. It is important that where possible the patient has the choice and thus can maintain control for as long as possible.

PRODUCTIVITY

It is important that patients feel productive throughout all stages of their disease. Many patients may have lost employment, the role that was associated with this, their income, their role as a parent, husband, wife or family member, the focus of their lives being disease-led. Becoming a patient can give rise to feelings of passivity and dependency.

An occupational therapist can provide some structure or a new role to encourage productivity. This ranges from advice on filling free time constructively following the loss of employment to helping the patient exchange his or her family role from breadwinner to housekeeper or if energy levels are severely limited, coordinating the shopping list for a home carer (Hensel *et al.*, 2002).

LEISURE

Leisure covers the activities from which a patient gains pleasure. Everyone's psychological well-being requires that they gain pleasure or enjoyment for some part of every day (Folkman and Greer, 2000). This is even more important for palliative care patients. In assessing their occupational components, care must be taken to address this area, ensuring that energy levels and functional abilities still allow pleasurable experiences (Unruh, 1997).

Leisure goals may become more difficult to achieve for the patient as disease progresses, but they remain of immense significance. It is important to recognize goals and where realistically possible help the patient to achieve them.

DAY CARE

For the purpose of this chapter specialist palliative day-care services will be discussed, however, it is recognized that general day-care services do provide a service for palliative care patients.

During recent years there has been an increase in specialist palliative day-care services with over 200 day-care services now available. Specialist palliative day-care services can be defined as 'Facilities that offer a range of opportunities for assessment and review of patients' needs and enable the provision of physical, psychological and social interventions within a context of social interaction, support and friendship' (House of Commons, 2004, p. 7).

Specialist palliative day-care services are able to provide a service to patients from professionals with specialized knowledge of palliative care conditions. Patients attending day care should have access to a range of clinicians such as:

- doctor
- nurse
- occupational therapist
- physiotherapist
- social worker
- psychologist
- dietitian
- speech and language therapist
- art therapist
- complementary therapists
- lymphoedema specialist
- chiropodist
- bereavement counsellor
- chaplain.

The core team of a multiprofessional team at a day-care unit would ideally consist of the first six clinicians. The extended team would involve various other professionals as mentioned above and volunteers who also play an important role in patient care. The multiprofessional team at a specialist day-care unit should aim to meet an individual's physical, emotional, spiritual and social needs. Having access to a wide range of professionals is hugely beneficial for the individual as care can be delivered in a holistic approach in one place (Spencer and Daniels, 1998).

Individuals are referred to palliative day-care units from a variety of sources, however this may vary within different localities. Typically, referrals are from professionals working in the community (e.g., district nurse, Macmillan nurse, allied health professionals), GP, consultant, relatives and the individual themselves. Patients attending day care will attend for various reasons depending on their individual need. This may range from symptom control, rehabilitation, respite, complementary therapies and the opportunity to talk to others in a similar situation. During the time spent at day care the patients needs' are regularly reviewed. This provides an opportunity to discuss whether the individual has benefited from the service, has a palliative care need and whether the service is meeting their needs. Although for most patients attendance ceases when the individual dies, some patients do recover and are discharged.

The occupational therapy role within a day-care setting is a valuable contribution to the multiprofessional team. However, it is important to remember that not all patients will wish to take part in an occupational therapy treatment programme and that their views should be respected. Patients wishing to have input from an occupational therapist may view this as an opportunity to improve their level of function (Low et al., 2005).

The occupational therapist role within the day-care unit may involve:

- assessment of needs with each individual to identify issues for treatment planning and setting up of treatment programme;
- observation of patients while undertaking functional/creative/leisure activities to highlight any unreported needs;
- assessment and review of patients' occupational performance in ADL tasks throughout their disease progression;
- assessment and treatment of cognitive and perceptual dysfunction;
- provision and demonstration of adaptive equipment such as toilet aids to enable independence;
- issue of small aids to enable independence in ADLs, e.g. adapted cutlery following a feeding assessment;
- splinting/referral for splinting by occupational therapy for prevention of postural deformities;
- provision of advice on energy conservation/fatigue management techniques;

- addressing wheelchair and pressure care seating issues;
- support of patient with psychological issues that may arise as a result of diagnosis, e.g. body image;
- rehabilitation sessions with physiotherapist to maintain/improve functional ability;
- advice on clothing and footwear;
- home assessment visits to review environmental issues or assess ADLs in patient's own environment;
- advise on appropriate accommodation in relation to current or projected needs.

The above points illustrate the wide range of skills an occupational therapist has to offer when working in a palliative day care setting. This skill base enables the occupational therapist to work holistically in a complex and challenging environment. The following case study illustrates this point:

CASE STUDY

Name: JS

Age: 78

Diagnosis: Cancer of the prostate, with spinal cord compression at T4, bone secondaries to his legs and spine. Prostate cancer was diagnosed in August 2001. The metastatic spread including spinal cord compression was diagnosed in August 2004.

Social situation: JS is a retired Civil Service Officer who held a senior position of considerable responsibility. Prior to day hospice attendance he had been an in-patient at the hospice. During this period, occupational therapy assistance was provided to assess the feasibility of return to his original accommodation and advice when viewing potential new accommodation. Occupational therapy also identified equipment essential for discharge home, arranged provision of specialist wheelchair and seating and worked closely with the physiotherapist to maximize safety in transfers.

JS's wife was very supportive but suffered from a chronic back condition. His daughter was also supportive but did not live locally. He had many friends in the area and enjoyed visiting a local social club prior to the onset of his spinal cord compression.

Professionals involved:

- palliative care occupational therapist;
- palliative care physiotherapist;
- palliative care social worker;
- day hospice team including complementary therapists (twice weekly visits);
- district nurse;
- home care manager.

Issues which were considered regarding JS's functional ability at time of transferring to the day hospice:

- supervision required for transfer between wheelchair, armchair, commode and bed using sliding board;
- able to propel wheelchair and access lounge, kitchen and bedroom independently;
- required 3 calls per day to assist with washing, dressing and use of commode;
- unable to access his balcony due to presence of step;
- unable to use bath or shower facilities at home;
- unable to transfer onto toilet;
- required assistance from daughter to transfer self and wheelchair into car;
- required assistance from daughter to access local facilities using wheelchair as wife unable to push wheelchair up steep slope at entrance to building.

Psycho-social considerations:

- JS was concerned about the additional stress and physical demands being placed on his wife due to his reduced level of independence.
- His wife was undergoing treatment for exacerbation of her back condition.
- JS felt frustrated by the difficulties he experienced with outdoor mobility.
- JS felt frustrated by being unable to access all areas of his home.

OCCUPATIONAL THERAPY INTERVENTION:

Clinical reasoning combined with observation up to this point of steady improvement in ability suggested that the most optimistic outcome of continued rehabilitation would be that JS would be able to take a few steps using a Zimmer frame and assistance.

Aims of treatment:

- to facilitate JS maximizing his independence in activities of daily living;
- to facilitate JS maximizing independence in outdoor mobility;
- to help reduce the physical and emotional demands on his wife;
- to provide ongoing advice and support as needs changed.

Occupational therapy goals: The following goals were agreed with JS with consideration of personal priorities for himself and his wife:

- to be able to access his balcony with minimal assistance;
- to be able to use his bath and shower facilities at home;
- to be able to transfer independently onto the toilet;
- to be able to transfer independently into the car and for his wife to be able to load the wheelchair;
- to be able to access local facilities and re-commence attendance at social club with minimal assistance.

Types of intervention:

- site visits to liaise with various agencies to identify ways of providing wheelchair access to balcony;
- joint occupational therapy and physiotherapy assessment and treatment sessions to improve ability and safety in transfers;
- provision of equipment following assessment and practice sessions in home environment to enable use of bath and over-bath shower at home;
- provision of equipment following assessment and practice sessions during hospice attendance and in home environment to enable independent use of toilet at home;
- practice sessions regarding transfer and liaison with local mobility equipment companies about ways of loading chair into car without his wife needing to lift;
- assistance in choosing appropriate powered wheelchair for outdoor use;
- liaison with other professionals about assistance with funding for powered wheelchair and associated pressure-relieving cushion.

SUMMARY:

Although intervention would continue with JS and his family, an evaluation took place to establish how his goals were being achieved. At that point, he now had a set of lightweight portable ramps, which his wife was able to put in place to allow him to access the balcony of his flat. These ramps could also be used to load his outdoor chair into his car. The transfer board was no longer required except occasionally for car transfers.

JS was able to use his bath and shower with minimal assistance but was awaiting minor modification of his care package. He no longer required his lunchtime care visit, as he was able to transfer on/off the commode or toilet independently and make the necessary adjustments to his clothing.

Assistance towards the purchase of an outdoor power wheelchair and pressure-relieving cushion was given by an organization related to his former employment. JS felt that his wife had benefited from his increased level of independence. In addition she enjoyed the free time that his twice weekly attendance at the day hospice gave her. She was aware of her eligibility for complementary therapy and family support services as additional coping strategies.

JS continued with his rehabilitation, which had been provided through regular sessions of occupational therapy and physiotherapy coordinated with complementary therapy and creative arts activities. He was able to stand independently from a high seat and walk a few steps using a Zimmer frame plus assistance.

ACTION POINTS

1. Discuss areas of research that are required into the role of the occupational therapist in palliative care, hospice or day care.
2. Explore the advantages and disadvantages of providing a rehabilitation service to patients in a palliative day-care setting or hospice.
3. Identify coping strategies and support mechanisms that you would use as an occupational therapist for working in a hospice environment when dealing with the terminally ill and the dying.

REFERENCES

Bray, J. (1997) Occupational therapy in hospices and day care, in *Occupational Therapy in Oncology and Palliative Care* (ed. J. Cooper), Whurr, London.

Dawson, S. and Barker, J. (1995) Hospice and palliative care: A delphi survey of occupational therapists' roles and training needs. *Australian Occupational Therapy Journal*, **42**(3), 119–27.

Department of Health (2000) *Cancer Plan*, HMSO, London.

Folkman, S. and Greer, S. (2000) Promoting psychological well-being in the face of serious illness: When theory, research and practice inform each other. *Psycho-Oncology*, **9**(1), 11–19.

Hensel, M., Egerer, G., Schneeweiss, A., Goldschmidt, H. and Ho, A. D. (2002) Quality of life and rehabilitation in social and professional life after autologous stem cell transplantation. *Annals of Oncology*, **13**(2), 209–17.

House of Commons (2004) *The House of Commons Health Committee Inquiry into Palliative Care – Submission of Evidence*, HMSO, London.

Low, J., Perry, R. and Wilkinson, S. (2005) A qualitative evaluation of the impact of palliative care day services: The experiences of patients, informal carers, day unit managers and volunteer staff. *Palliative Medicine*, **19**(1), 65–70.

Lyons, M., Orozovic, N., Davis, J. and Newman, J. (2002) Doing-being-becoming: Occupational experiences of persons with life-threatening illnesses. *American Journal of Occupational Therapy*, **56**(3), 285–95.

MacLaren, J. (1996) Rehabilitation through advocacy and empowerment. *British Journal of Occupational Therapy*, **3**(9), 492–7.

National Council for Hospice and Specialist Palliative Care Services (1995) *Statement of Definitions*, NCHSPCS, London.

National Council for Hospice and Specialist Palliative Care Services (2002) *Fulfilling Lives: Rehabilitation in palliative care*, NCHSPCS, London.

Reed, K. and Sanderson, S. (1988) *Concepts of Occupational Therapy*, 2nd edn, Williams & Wilkins, Baltimore, MD.

Soderback, I. and Paulsson, E. H. (1997) A needs assessment for referral to occupational therapy: Nurses' judgement in acute cancer care. *Cancer Nurse*, **20**(4), 267–73.

Spencer, D. J. and Daniels, L. E. (1998) Day hospice care: A review of the literature. *Palliative Medicine*, **12**(4), 219–29.

Townsend, E., Stanton, S. and Law, M. (1997) *Enabling Occupation: An occupational therapy perspective*, Canadian Association of Occupational Therapists, Ottawa.

Unruh, A. M. (1997) Spirituality and occupation: Garden musings and the Himalayan Blue Poppy. *Canadian Journal of Occupational Therapy*, **64**(1), 156–60.

Vrkljan, B. H. and Miller-Polgar, J. (2001) Meaning of occupational engagement in life-threatening illness: A qualitative pilot project. *Canadian Journal of Occupational Therapy*, **68**(4), 237–46.

Wilcock, A., Chelin, M. and Hall, M. (1997) The relationship between occupational balance and health: A pilot study. *Occupational Therapy International*, **4**(1), 17–30.

World Health Organization (2002) *National Cancer Control Programmes: Policies and managerial guidelines*, 2nd edn. WHO, Geneva.

12 The Use of Creativity as a Psychodynamic Activity

KATHRYN BOOG

THE PSYCHODYNAMIC APPROACH

In occupational therapy, creative activity used as a form of communication can empower patients to express their innermost thoughts and feelings non-verbally. Both the creative process and the object produced as the outcome are of equal importance in the path leading towards self-actualization and closure at the end of life.

An examination of the literature supports the view that being given a life-limiting prognosis raises important issues for palliative care patients where they review and reflect on their lives – they feel the need to have achievements acknowledged and to leave behind tangible reminders of themselves and their lives.

As life draws to an end, people can feel a sense of urgency to bring certain aspects of their lives to a conclusion by addressing, and hopefully resolving to their satisfaction, issues that have caused them a degree of angst. These may have been pushed into the background and not adequately dealt with at the time but are now bubbling to the surface at the end of life, making emotional closure difficult to achieve. The successful management of symptoms often seems to be the trigger for this appraisal, reflecting Maslow's (1968) pyramid of hierarchy and the higher human needs for creativity and personal growth (Connell, 1989; Kennett, 2000). At this transitional phase in people's lives, we are acknowledging their life experience, abilities and achievements, while at the same time being aware of their impending deterioration and approaching death (Bye, 1998). Creative activity can be a catalyst in this dichotomous process, as an aid to communication and assessment as well as a means of expression and connection with others at a time when this can be difficult. It is a useful adjunct to pharmacological symptom management but for the purposes of this chapter, the main emphasis will be on its application when dealing with emotional and spiritual issues, facilitating the release of these feelings and the conclusion of related unfinished business.

Occupational Therapy in Oncology and Palliative Care. Edited by J. Cooper
© 2006 John Wiley & Sons Ltd

ASSESSMENT

Management of pain, breathlessness and fatigue can be a complex issue due to individuals' personal experience of these symptoms and their ability to deal with their illness. Solutions in this case need to be multifaceted and assessment should include the following:

- viewing the relationship between physical ability to function and psychological, social and spiritual influences on that ability (SIGN, 2000);
- examining life roles. These are individually interpreted and influenced by culture and society and have unique meaning to each person;
- exploring goals and ambitions related to these life roles;
- identifying remaining strengths and capabilities rather than focusing on deteriorating health;
- refocusing on important issues for the patient and family;
- constant reassessing to address changing needs.

A decreased performance level in creative activity will be an indicator of a lower level of occupational function in activities of daily living and therefore a stimulus for reassessment of the situation (Holland, 1984).

THE THERAPEUTIC RELATIONSHIP

The importance of the therapeutic relationship when dealing with psychological, emotional and spiritual issues cannot be underestimated if a true picture of patients is to be drawn, and their real aims are to be revealed. Rogers' (1961) three core conditions of empathy, unconditional positive regard and congruence will encourage a facilitative environment in which the creative process can be the means of achieving self-actualization. The individuals' needs, desires, hopes and fears, goals and ambitions and feelings of loss may be revealed and the holistic overview will enable development of a strategy to enhance their lifestyle and make it as rewarding as possible. A re-evaluation of occupational performance and the realignment of new life goals will allow for continued productivity and competency and maintain integrity, self-esteem and dignity. By highlighting the patients' abilities rather than their disabilities and offering alternative, achievable choices of activity, they can still feel able to participate in life roles and decision-making.

Sitting quietly and **being with** the patient during the creative process will allow the therapist to observe behaviour, while **working alongside** during the activity will also facilitate the development of a therapeutic, trusting relationship. Patients present not only with their illness, but with all of their life's baggage in tow, including previous illnesses, relationship issues, social, spiritual and emotional components, which all bring to bear on the situation.

The occupational therapist needs to be responsive and open to both verbal and non-verbal cues that the patient may intentionally or unintentionally give out and be prepared to act on these, perhaps using counselling techniques to direct the conversation. However, caution needs to be exerted in order that the proverbial 'can of worms' is not opened without the means to deal with it. It is also important to mention here the therapeutic use of self which will be influenced by the therapist's own beliefs and coping strategies (Bye, 1998; Rahman, 2000).

USING COUNSELLING SKILLS

Patients need to be motivated to achieve goals and we should be aware that some may focus on their physical difficulties and hide behind their inability to function as a way to avoid confronting emotional issues such as anxiety, anger, fear and associated loss. In order to have a better understanding of the goals and ambitions of these patients, counselling techniques may be useful.

By using these skills to enhance the psychodynamic approach in occupational therapy, the occupational therapist can enable the patient to identify and deal appropriately with end-of-life issues. This is not a counselling session, but merely using the approach as a tool to help patients make sense of what is going on for them and decide on an acceptable course of action. A suggested technique might be to start with an open conversational question – 'How are you today?' Then use a mixture of open and closed questions, review and clarify, follow and lead, and allow silences.

COMMUNICATION ISSUES

People with communication problems are very vulnerable, especially at times of transition – moving from home to hospice, for example: they need their carers to know what is important to them in order that they may feel comfortable and safe. Communication charts should be made available perhaps in consultation with a speech therapist, and for those with cognitive difficulties, life story books provide a useful adjunct to medical notes. These can be used not only for communication, but also for meaningful interaction with that person. A communication file might also be considered. This is a highly personalized book, which is similar to a life story and contains information about the patient's wants, likes and dislikes, family, etc. It allows those coming into contact with and caring for the patient to have an understanding of that person's needs and wishes.

An extension of this idea is a communication diary which can be used as a link between, for example, day hospice and home when the patient's family want to find out what has been happening during the day. It allows the patient to remain autonomous and facilitates the conversation at home.

Rapport between the occupational therapist and patient and the quality of the therapeutic alliance is one of the major factors that will reflect the depth of exchange. Bye (1998) presents the idea that the quality of the interaction between patient and therapist has equal importance with achievement of goals.

Creativity can be used as a non-threatening means of interaction, creating a more relaxed atmosphere where the patient feels he can share thoughts and feelings with the therapist. The lack of eye contact, when concentrating on the project, can make it easier for the patient to express himself. The object being produced can work as a catalyst in the process, making dialogue easier by transferring the emphasis from the therapist to the activity. By working together on a shared activity, the interaction becomes less clinical and will allow a greater depth of conversation between the two, allowing an insight into the person behind the illness (Perrin, 2001).

The symbolic relevance of creative activity can prove to be a very useful tool for both needs assessment and treatment strategy in this setting. Working together on creative activities allows for concentration on something other than illness, and the relaxed atmosphere seems to encourage a return to 'normal' social conversation. Through careful use of counselling skills in this situation, the therapist can gently encourage patients to reveal something of themselves. It is important to be aware that sometimes patients will give socially desirable answers, so observation of body language is a useful tool in the assessment process. Non-verbal communication can give useful clues as to what the patient is really saying/meaning as words and body language often conflict.

ROLES AND GOAL SETTING

Inability to participate in those familiar occupations which define the individual's role can make adaptation to the changing circumstances physically, psychologically or socially difficult. Relinquishing occupational roles can affect feelings of worth and the person's sense of dignity, and so constant re-assessment of functional ability is important to address changing needs. A re-evaluation of occupational performance leading to the realignment of new life goals, no matter how small, will allow the patient to remain productive and competent, encouraging motivation and maintaining their integrity and self-esteem.

People who can no longer actively maintain their life roles still need to feel satisfied and productive through occupational engagement. By revealing their strengths and concentrating on these rather than their weaknesses, and by working with their abilities and suggesting other acceptable and attainable goals, they can still feel they have a role to play. Creative activities can be a means of fulfilling these needs, of moving forward to the future, and of offering hope. In a discussion paper evaluating health promotion as a quality of life issue in palliative care, vanderPloeg (2001) states that, 'Individuals are not only adaptive but also have the potential to transcend difficulties and create new patterns of behaviour enabling continuation of a meaningful and satisfying existence.' In parallel with all other areas of therapeutic intervention, it is vitally important to be aware of patients' goals and ambitions in order for these activities to have meaning and purpose. Only then are we moving away from the reductionist model and treating the whole person (Holder, 2001).

NARRATIVE

Life stories are valuable resources in occupational therapy because they are personal interpretations of people's occupational participation throughout their life course (Wicks and Whiteford, 2003). A knowledge of personal life experience, relationships and previous coping patterns can give a strong indication of how people will cope with a transitional phase in their life, such as death and dying (Blair, 2000; Rahman, 2000).

The assessment process will be greatly enhanced by using a narrative approach that will allow the occupational therapist to empathize with patients by entering into their lived experience. This can be used to help identify feelings and needs and explore goals and ambitions. By reflecting on past life issues that are important to the patient and that can have significant bearing on present coping strategies, both occupational therapist and patient can design a programme together that will allow the remaining life to be lived as constructively as the patient wishes. Mattingly (1991) describes this as the therapist helping create a therapeutic story that becomes a meaningful short story in the larger life story of the patient.

Narrative, as used in the psychodynamic approach, is recommended by Burton (1991) to locate the illness within that person's life story. This provides the opportunity for patients to reflect on past experiences and to re-situate themselves within their present view of their life. In this way reactions to current events and the resulting emotional responses may be better understood. The subjective nature of the patient's perspectives will give a realistic insight into their personal experiences and their feelings regarding these.

The narrative approach will enable the occupational therapist to discover meanings attached to particular occupations for individuals and how they express themselves through these occupations. An understanding of these will ensure the choice of meaningful creative activity supporting the patient through this period of transition.

Although the person's account of events is generally subjective and therefore may not reflect an accurate picture of events, the account does portray the patients' perceived experience of that situation and the truth as they see it. The relationship between the meaning of various occupations and how they fit into their role should thus be made clearer.

For some patients, formalizing this type of narrative can be a means not only of communication but also of affirming life – of seeking out positives and underlining personhood and identity, improving self-esteem and creating feelings of value and worth. 'The life review, Janus-like, involves facing death as well as looking back' (Butler, 1963).

Life stories can serve as memory albums for families, where narratives can be shared and recorded for perpetuity and may also contain letters and cards of final farewell.

CASE STUDY

As Peter neared the end of life, he recalled happy memories of his daughter's childhood and enjoyed telling her stories during her visits. Over a period of time, he realized that although he could recall many of these little vignettes in great detail, his daughter was hearing them as if for the first time. The memories and the stories were precious and they both wanted to have a permanent record of them and so Peter asked if he could dictate them and have some help to create a little story book of his daughter's childhood. He was extremely fatigued and could only work for short periods at a time, but slowly, the project developed. Photographs were produced by members of the family and scanned on to the pages, and the life story book produced was filled with stories of love and pride with just a sprinkling of humour. A fitting last gift.

CREATIVE ACTIVITIES

The creative process is used in occupational therapy to bring about change in people and in their ability to deal with the world around them. As well as the significance of the object produced in this process, equal importance is attached to the more intangible outcomes. This includes the satisfaction gained at being able to express feelings, improved self-esteem and worthiness and a feeling of return of some control into peoples' lives. People's relationships, roles, ambitions and goals can also be affected as a direct consequence of these cathartic changes, resulting in a return of self-respect and self-confidence. Patients are often surprised at their abilities to learn new activities at this time and this self-development can lead to an reawakening of self-identity and, ultimately, self-fulfilment.

The mere act of creation can release previously withheld emotions that are directed towards, and into, the object, so privacy in which to work is essential here. Creative art can be merely for enjoyment purposes to begin with, but very often develops into a cathartic experience for the patient. Card making, writing poetry, silk painting, glass painting, collage, stencilling and woodwork are examples of activities that have been developed in this way, and which facilitate not only emotional expression, but also a sense of continuity that is very important to people whose lives are limited. Continuity and being remembered can be achieved by the making of gifts and also by photographing/scanning projects such as glass paintings, silk paintings or collage work and using the images to create notelets, calendars or cards which can then either be used by the patient or sold in the hospice shop.

CASE STUDY

An elderly woman, who had always wanted to paint with acrylics, was given a painting-by-numbers set by her sister in Australia. When she had finished the work, we discussed how the snow scene could be scanned and then printed on to cards and individual greetings printed on the word processor to make personalized Christmas cards. She was delighted with the results, as was her sister who was able to see how beautifully the picture had been painted.

Life-limiting disease can result in a whole range of negative feelings within a family unit. There can be anger and resentment at the changes in responsibilities and roles and the myriad losses involved. Past relationship difficulties may re-emerge, along with a subsequent wish to reconnect with people. There may be a need to express a variety of emotions and so effect closure.

When any or all of these issues are compounded by anger, this serves to create a situation where family members are alienated one from the other, resulting in hurt and a needless lack of communication (Gammage et al., 1976).

We don't just receive people who are reaching the end of their lives; we receive families where ties have been unhealthy for years, and which now reveal their weakness and deficiencies. Because nothing can remain hidden when there's so little time left, and when everything that was acting as a screen suddenly looks so flimsy. When one's intimacy is rooted in another person's and one feels a rapport, silence can feel like a benediction. But not for those separated by a trench.

(de Hennezel, 1997)

Creative activities can facilitate the re-connection of positive emotions by allowing the patient free expression of his innermost feelings in a controlled and acceptable way, leading the way towards emotional closure in the preparation for death. Patients may make this connection with others in the form of creative art and creative writing.

Cognitive difficulties, literacy or speech problems are not barriers to creativity as, for any of the activities requiring the written word, the occupational therapist can be scribe. Perrin and May (2000) strongly advise those of us involved with people's health and welfare to give urgent consideration to the fostering of creativity. Using creative activities to transcend the hurdle of cognitive difficulties will allow people to interact with and feel part of the group. In this situation, the activity can be a catalyst for communication between the individual and the rest of the group.

Using prepared or computer-generated images means that those who consider themselves not to be artistic can choose pictures that they feel are representative of their own ideas and allow them to still participate fully in the activity (Williams, 2002).

When it is no longer possible to achieve physical control or independence, control at a cognitive/psychological level can be emphasized. Patients can still make decisions about personal matters and express their individuality through artwork. Again the occupational therapist can be the patient's hands to allow the patient to use his imagination and ideas freely. People who can no longer communicate either verbally or by pointing can direct the work by eye movements.

Of course, the core skill of occupational therapists, the ability to analyse an activity and make that activity attainable to the patient is crucial for a successful outcome. This will allow people to gain pleasure from the activities and want to continue, encouraging psychological well-being through the continued building of self-esteem and worth.

In a qualitative study of groupwork at an Australian hospice, it was found that in a group situation, the occupational therapist could facilitate 'interaction, sharing, caring, remembering and, thus, decrease feelings of helplessness and isolation' (Dawson, 1993). Patients begin to feel a sense of belonging to the group as they begin to communicate with the others and become aware of each other's needs and some have even described it as 'like being in a family' (Mee and Sumsion, 2001).

Card making is a very acceptable medium to the patient, as a means of expressing themself. It can bring about feelings of relief at being able to release previously withheld emotions, helping in stress and anxiety management. While the therapist is working alongside the patient to prepare the artwork for the cover, the opportunity can be used to develop the therapeutic relationship and find out more about the recipient of the card and what exactly the patient would like to say. Focusing on the artwork will allow sensitive issues to be raised and perhaps discussed. In fact, using an activity like this as a catalyst can free the patient to discuss or avoid certain issues as the mood dictates. Collage, silk painting, embossing and digital imagery are just some of the ways that a design can be developed for the card.

The appearance of the finished design is very important to patients, and a piece of work that is acceptable to them and that pleases them will boost their self-esteem, give them a sense of achievement and motivate them to continue (Thompson and Blair, 1998).

People find it much easier to use written words to express themselves than to speak them, and the content of the written material inside the card is often developed as a short piece of creative writing. In a qualitative study exploring the relationship between creative writing and mental well-being, Jensen and Blair attributed the therapeutic reasons for this to 'the resolution of unconscious conflicts, the creation of a transitional space, and as a productive and purposeful task' (Jensen and Blair, 1997).

Poetry writing can also enable patients to express things that they find difficult if not impossible to say aloud. Being able to write about emotions and to transfer these feelings and dreams on to paper can be a comforting experience (Connell, 1989). The message can be of love or hope, or of sadness and hurt, but whatever the reason for writing the poem, it will allow the experience to be a shared one. Again, it will also be a tangible memory of that person and can be made into a card or picture as a gift for a loved one or pinned up in their room.

ARTWORK

Artwork can be described as making memories and as a mark of one's existence (Perrin, 2001) and thereby 'establishing a sense of one's past, present, and future' (Kennett, 2000). It is very important to emphasize to patients that their work will be treated confidentially and that no one will see any of it except the patient and the occupational therapist. It is the patient's property and the importance of this must be acknowledged at the outset. This will further underline the trusting relationship described previously, and encourage the sharing of information crucial to the success of the project.

Some people will require a lot of help with their project, involving a considerable amount of time devoted to the preparation, execution and finishing off of the work. At all times, patients must feel that it is their work and that the decisions about creating the object are all theirs. When it is no longer physically possible for people to do things for themselves, it is still important that they are involved in decision making. Saying, 'You are the one with the ideas and my hands can carry them out for you' is often enough to support the feeling of still being in control for the patient. Respect for the piece of work is also very important, handling it carefully, and storing it safely, will attach a value to it. The object can be the focus for emotions, a tangible representation of someone's feelings. It may be the last gift they ever give someone, a final birthday or Christmas present, a thank you for help and support. It will be a reminder to the recipient of a life, a relationship, a parent perhaps that a child will barely remember, and must be handled as the precious gift that it is.

The emotions invoked may be a trigger to the release of thoughts and memories relating to difficult periods in the patient's life, and the team approach is essential here. Perhaps the clinical psychologist will need to be consulted for their expertise in this area.

CONSTRAINTS

As with any activity undertaken by these patients, there are certain constraints that will inhibit their participation:

- physical discomfort, due to pain, dyspnoea, nausea, etc.;
- depleted energy levels and lethargy;
- attentional fatigue, or poor concentration;
- emotional trauma;
- lack of motivation;
- time.

Continuous monitoring of the activities in order to keep them within that person's range of abilities will ensure success, along with planning, pacing and prioritizing and may include relaxation sessions using guided imagery.

CASE STUDY

A 35-year-old woman with recently diagnosed, but terminal, throat cancer had so many things she wanted to do before she died, but was lacking the energy to be able to think clearly and prioritize her goals. At her first visit to the day centre, she agreed to try relaxation and requested that we use the image of a beach. She was given a tape to use at home and on her next visit reported that her husband had joined her and that afterwards they had discussed the pictures that it had conjured up for them. They had both been using images of a beach holiday that they had shared, and the experience stimulated discussion and reminiscence of the many beach holidays they had had as a couple and also as a family with their young children. Would the children remember those happy times with their mother? They had photographs, but stories, in the words of their mother, of experiences they had shared were something that the couple were keen to pursue. With help from the therapist, they were encouraged to make a memory album for the children, using travel brochures, photos, small mementoes and tales of their holidays as a family, written in their mother's words.

DOING AND BECOMING – A TRANSITION

Life roles are individually interpreted and influenced by culture and social activity. Acknowledging and accepting lost roles and adjusting to new ones can be described as viewing the meaning of who we are from a different perspective (Rahman, 2000).

In order to adjust to these changing life roles, people need to make the transition from a doing person to a being person. This will be the result of a voyage of self-discovery in which the patients, through reflection and an exploration of themselves during the psychodynamic process, will have the opportunity to 'develop, change, grow and be better' – and become (Lyons *et al.*, 2002).

For those unable to participate physically in the transition process, patients can still influence their activities and exercise choice by directing carers to carry out their wishes. With creative activities, by offering a choice of materials, designs, words, etc., patients can still feel that the act of creation is their own.

SPIRITUALITY – IS IT ADDRESSED CREATIVELY?

In attempting to define spirituality, various articles suggest it is about:

- searching for meaning, value and purpose – hope for the future;
- belonging and connecting with others and relationships – a sense of self-worth and identity.

The anxiety, agitation and guilt that some patients experience can result in feelings of loss at being unable to achieve these goals.

When we enter the patient's world through the processes of assessment, watching for non-verbal cues and listening to their narrative of their life's experiences, we are trying to hear what they are really saying. Only then can we begin to empathize with them and help in the discovery of who and where they are, and their ambitions for the future. In treatment planning, the patient's desire to respond to emotional issues by leaving behind keepsakes can be addressed creatively. The human desire to remind others of one's existence, to leave behind tangible memories and effect emotional closure in the preparation for death, can be achieved.

'The search for meaning, for something in which to trust, may be expressed in many ways, direct or indirect, in metaphor or in silence, in gesture or in symbol or, perhaps most of all, in art and the unexpected potential for creativity at the end of life' (Saunders, 1996).

In summary, the value of creativity in palliative care can be viewed as a means to:

- enhance communication in the assessment and reassessment process;
- encourage people to reflect back to the past and to situate their present circumstances in their life story;
- allow emotional expression, both verbal and non-verbal (Thompson and Blair, 1998);
- create gifts to express emotions and to ensure remembrance of the person, and therefore affirmation of their future – *I will leave this behind and people will remember me when they see it*;
- deal with unfinished business, both practical and emotional;
- effect emotional closure;
- return the sense of control, and therefore hope and self-esteem;
- allow patients to feel they are making a contribution to society, instead of always receiving, as with reminiscence and creative art, writing.

REFERENCES

Blair, S. E. E. (2000) The centrality of occupation during life transitions. *British Journal of Occupational Therapy*, **63**(5), 231–7.

Burton, M. V. (1991) Counselling in routine care: A client-centred approach, in *Cancer Patient Care: Psychosocial treatment methods* (ed. M. Watson), BPS Books, Cambridge.

Butler, R. N. (1963) The life review: An interpretation of reminiscence in the aged. *Psychiatry*, February 26, 65–76.

Bye, R. A. (1998) When clients are dying: Occupational therapists' perspectives. *Occupational Therapy Journal of Research*, **18**(1), 3–22.

Connell, H. (1989) Promoting creative expression. *Nursing Times*, **85**(15), 52–4.

Dawson, S. (1993) The role of occupational therapy groups in an Australian hospice. *The American Journal of Hospice and Palliative Care*, **10**(4), 13–17.

de Hennezel, M. (1997) *Intimate Death: How the dying teach us to live*, Warner, London.

Gammage, S. L., McMahon, P. S. and Shanahan, P. M. (1976) The occupational therapist and terminal illness: Learning to cope with death. *American Journal of Occupational Therapy*, **30**(5), 294–9.

Holder, V. (2001) The use of creative activities within occupational therapy. *British Journal of Occupational Therapy*, **64**(2), 103–5.

Holland, A. E. (1984) Occupational therapy and day care for the terminally Ill. *British Journal of Occupational Therapy*, **47**(11), 345–8.

Jensen, C. M. and Blair, S. E. E. (1997) Rhyme and reason: The relationship between creative writing and mental wellbeing. *British Journal of Occupational Therapy*, **60**(12), 525–30.

Kennett, C. E. (2000) Participation in a creative arts project can foster hope in a hospice day centre. *Palliative Medicine*, **14**(5), 419–25.

Lyons, M., Orozovic, N., Davis, J. and Newman, J. (2002) Doing-being-becoming: Occupational experiences of persons with life-threatening illnesses. *American Journal of Occupational Therapy*, **56**(3), 285–95.

Maslow, A. (1968) *Towards a psychology of being*, 2nd edn, Van Nostrand, Toronto.

Mattingly, C. (1991) The narrative nature of clinical reasoning. *The American Journal of Occupational Therapy*, **45**(11), 998–1005.

Mee, J. and Sumsion, T. (2001) Mental health clients confirm the motivating power of occupation. *British Journal of Occupational Therapy*, **64**(3), 121–8.

Perrin, T. (2001) Don't despise the fluffy bunny: A reflection from practice. *British Journal of Occupational Therapy*, **64**(3), 129–34.

Perrin, T. and May, H. (2000) *Wellbeing in Dementia: An occupational approach for therapists and carers*, Churchill Livingstone, London.

Rahman, H. (2000) Journey of providing care in hospice: Perspectives of occupational therapists. *Qualitative Health Research*, **10**(6), 806–18.

Rogers, C. R. (1961) *On Becoming a Person*, Constable, London.

Saunders, C. (1996) Into the valley of the shadow of death. *British Medical Journal*, **313**(7072), 1599–1601.

SIGN (2000) *Control of Pain in Patients with Cancer. Guideline no. 44*, Scottish Intercollegiate Guidelines Network, Edinburgh.

Thompson, M. and Blair, S. E. E. (1998) Creative arts in occupational therapy: Ancient history or contemporary practice? *Occupational Therapy International*, **5**(1), 49–65.

vanderPloeg, W. (2001) Health promotion in palliative care: An occupational perspective. *Australian Occupational Therapy Journal*, **48**(1), 45–8.

Wicks, A. and Whiteford, G. (2003) Value of life stories in occupation-based research. *Australian Occupational Therapy Journal*, **50**(2), 86–91.

Williams, B. (2002) Teaching through artwork in terminal care. *European Journal of Palliative Care*, **9**(1), 34–6.

13 Measuring Occupational Therapy Outcomes in Cancer and Palliative Care

GAIL EVA

Evaluating the services we provide is important. We need to ensure that our patients are receiving the best possible care. National policy (Department of Health, 2000), guidelines (NICE, 2004), and the individual organizations in which we work, require that we are able to demonstrate that patients' needs are being met.

Occupational therapists working in cancer and palliative care must be able to evaluate their own services and contribute to multiprofessional evaluations for a number of good reasons, for example:

- to demonstrate that the interventions provided are effective;
- to guide the development of services;
- to monitor the impact of service developments and changes to practice;
- to show patients and their families that they are making progress.

There are a range of ways in which this can be achieved, measuring outcomes being just one option among many. It will often be useful to incorporate a range of indicators in an evaluation. Some alternatives to consider would be:

- collecting and presenting **base-line service data**, for example, the number of patients referred, the number of patients seen, demographic details of patients, the speed of response to referrals, the number of home visits undertaken, and the type and cost of equipment provided;
- conducting **service audits** to demonstrate that the standards set are being achieved, for example, that all palliative care patients are seen within 24 hours of referral;
- carrying out **patient satisfaction surveys** can be useful if the survey is well designed and carefully implemented (for a very good review of patient satisfaction measures in palliative care, see Aspinal et al., 2003);

Occupational Therapy in Oncology and Palliative Care. Edited by J. Cooper
© 2006 John Wiley & Sons Ltd

- using a data collection tool or structure that will enable the **measurement of the outcomes** of an intervention. The focus of this chapter will be on this aspect of service evaluation.

OUTCOME MEASURES

Outcome measures are useful tools for providing objective evidence of the value of an intervention. An 'outcome' is the change that has occurred as a result of that intervention. Put fairly simply: a patient is finding it increasingly difficult to look after herself independently, but after a fatigue management programme becomes able to plan and pace daily activities. Being able to quantify this change in some way will provide us with good evidence for the effectiveness of the programme.

This is easily said, but perhaps not quite so effortlessly done. Measuring the outcomes of occupational therapy interventions in palliative care has proved problematic (Norris, 1999), and occupational therapists have struggled to identify appropriate measures (HOPE, 1999). However, with forethought and planning, it is possible to gather data on outcomes that can be useful in a variety of ways.

THE NATURE OF OUTCOMES IN CANCER AND PALLIATIVE CARE: IMPROVEMENT VERSUS DETERIORATION

In selecting appropriate measures, it is important to consider what counts as a meaningful outcome. The Canadian Association of Occupational Therapists (1997) take the primary role of occupational therapy to be enabling occupation, where occupation includes all activities of daily life: taking care of yourself, having fun, and being productively involved in family and community living. Although there is acknowledgement in the occupational therapy literature that the attainment of perfect health and independence is not the goal of occupational therapy intervention, there is, none the less, an emphasis on restoring and improving a person's occupational performance, and outcome measures such as the Assessment of Motor and Process Skills (AMPS) and the Functional Independence Measure (FIM) reflect this. Sources of further information on all measures referred to can be found at the end of the chapter.

Many of the cancer patients who are referred to occupational therapy will have disabilities resulting from advanced disease, and interventions aimed at dramatic improvements in function and independence will not be appropriate. The selection of measures will need to take this into account.

In a thought-provoking paper, Bye (1998, p. 4) describes the difficulty faced by occupational therapists working in palliative care: 'People with terminal illness do not fit [a rehabilitative approach] because they lose roles and eventually withdraw from society . . . People who are terminally ill progressively deteriorate in terms of their functional independence, often require a significant amount of care from others and do not go on to live productive lives. They die.' In order to be meaningful, the focus of occupational therapy must be on valuing the life that a person has left to live, identifying the occupations and roles that remain important, and enabling patients to participate in these.

MULTIPROFESSIONAL TEAMWORKING AND OUTCOMES

The importance of good multiprofessional teamwork is central to the effective delivery of palliative care (NCHSPCS, 1999; Department of Health, 2000; NICE, 2004). Patients with life-threatening illnesses face a multitude of issues, and are highly individual in the ways that they seek support. To be able to understand adequately, and to intervene in the psychological, physical and spiritual areas of life requires a wide range of skills, and, consequently, patient care is best provided by a number of different professionals with their own areas of expertise. It may not be realistic or practical to separate occupational therapy intervention from the total package, and outcome measures that reflect the contribution of a team may be more useful than profession-specific measures. Of course, this approach may not identify the specific contribution of occupational therapy, but it might be more realistic and achievable to measure group outcomes. Examples of general measures that have been shown to work effectively in palliative care include the Palliative care Outcomes Scale (POS) and the Schedule for the Evaluation of Individualised Quality of Life – Direct Weighting (SEIQoL-DW).

ORGANIZATIONAL ISSUES

The way in which outcomes are measured creates an agenda for the planning and delivery of services. Organizational outcomes that are measured through, for example, length of stay and readmission rates, need to be incorporated with the patients' perspectives on the service they receive. Excluding the patient's voice in deciding on what constitutes a meaningful outcome risks providing services that are not relevant to those who use them. While there are clear benefits in measuring outcomes, there is also a need for recognition of the limits of information obtained in this way. Too great a reliance on outcomes data in planning services risks a narrow, prescriptive approach to patient care, and can be misused to justify cost cutting and rationing (Grahame-Smith, 1995; Long and Harrison, 1996).

OCCUPATIONAL THERAPISTS' IDEAS ON OUTCOMES

In the literature, occupational therapists describe a number of desirable outcomes for cancer and palliative care patients resulting from occupational therapy. Some examples follow:

- Patients are able to maintain continuity of usual daily activity, which allows a sense of normality and order during a time of change and disruption (Bye, 1998).
- Patients are able to gain control – both physical and psychological – over their lives, in areas such as decision-making, setting goals, privacy and daily activities (Lloyd and Coggles, 1990; Bye, 1998).
- Patients' environments are safe, and both patients and carers have knowledge of resources to promote a sense of safety and security (Bye, 1998).
- Patients and their families are assisting in achieving 'closure' in aspects of their lives (Hasselkus, 1993; Bye, 1998).

PATIENTS' PERCEPTIONS OF OUTCOMES

In a study to determine patients' perceptions of occupational therapy outcomes, Eva (2001) suggests that occupational therapy intervention is important to patients. Patients should be encouraged either to try activities that they may not have had the confidence to attempt on their own, or that might not have occurred to them. A patient talks about being introduced to watercolour painting:

> It's their encouragement to try things. Even though I can't do all of it myself in the way that I used to, it's still satisfying. It's started me off again, doing things at home. I've gone out and bought paints and an easel. I was feeling so frustrated before. It's been really good. I think with cancer patients particularly, it's important, particularly if you're disabled, because then obviously you can't get out like you normally would, you can't drive. There's so much . . . so many things you can't do. You have to be really encouraged to try new things.

There should be a broad spectrum of occupation, looking at activities that are pleasurable in addition to those that are necessary. The provision of equipment to facilitate independence was a vital and valued aspect of occupational therapy, but when this was not coupled with meeting patients' emotional and psychological needs, it was regarded as limited in scope:

I needed one of those devices to help put a stocking on my foot. She got me that, you know, an aid. And then the next thing, in the afternoon, we were baking. She combines the two things whereas other occupational therapists I've met haven't, they don't do that. They just see to your needs, your personal needs, and that's it. The OTs who have been the most helpful, they've looked across a big spectrum. It's looked across right from needs to pleasure.

There should be a resource for practical information related to living with a disability, and also for prompt advice on and supply of equipment and adaptations:

Well, I've felt that there is somebody out there that cares. There is somebody else I can speak to if I need anything. I know there's somebody on the end of a phone to help if I'm having difficulty managing things. I've been luckier than most. It's always been there when I needed it, and they've done it immediately.

Patients should be enabled to continue with valued roles. Patients valued being able to contribute to family and social life:

Take Sunday afternoon. My family took the dogs out on a long walk. I stayed behind, obviously. And after a bit, I thought, well, I'll start the tea, so we wouldn't be waiting around at the time they came home, an hour and a half later. I have the stool there, so it was easy for me to sit and peel a few potatoes and do a few vegetables, and I could put the meat in the oven. I had the confidence to know I could do it. And there was everything cooking when they came in, and they were thrilled. It was just right. I felt so good that I could do it.

INITIAL CONSIDERATIONS ON MEASURING OUTCOMES

The following is a list of some questions that might help in the process of deciding on a measure. It is important to remember that the single perfect measure, suitable for all applications, does not exist. All measures have their strengths and weaknesses.

- Start by being clear and specific about *why* you want to measure outcomes. You may need to back up a bid for funding, or it may be required as part of a departmental audit. Having a specific project or question to answer makes it much easier to identify what data will be required, rather than starting with the vague gesture that 'I need to know that I'm making a difference.'
- Who are the results intended to be useful to? Who will you need to communicate them to, and how? Do you need to show an individual patient that he or she is making progress, or will you need data from a large number of cases to present to the management of your organization?

- How much time do you have to spend on the project? What resources are available to you?
- What outcomes are you aiming to achieve? What do you anticipate that patients will gain as a result of your intervention? Make a list of these domains. They may be general to a group of patients, for example, 'to reduce levels of anxiety for patients undergoing a relaxation training programme', or specific to an individual patient, for example, 'to enable Mrs A to prepare meals for her family'. Knowing what your intended outcomes are will make it easier to identify appropriate measures. Outcomes which are generalizable to a group will be amenable to generic scaling methods such as POS, whereas those specific to an individual will require individualized measures, such as goal setting or the Schedule for the Evaluation of Individualised Quality of Life – Direct Weighting (SEIQoL-DW).
- Have the staff who are going to use the outcome measure had adequate training in its use, and is everyone involved committed to the project? Are the benefits of the additional work – because collecting and analysing data **will** involve additional work – clear to all?

SOME POSSIBLE OCCUPATIONAL THERAPY MEASURES

THE CANADIAN OCCUPATIONAL PERFORMANCE MEASURE (COPM)

The Canadian Occupational Performance Measure (COPM) is based on the Canadian Occupational Performance Model of occupational therapy practice, a model which is particularly suited to palliative care as it recognizes the influence of physical, socio-cultural, mental and spiritual domains on a person's occupational performance (Law et al., 1994). The COPM uses a client-centred approach. It measures client-identified problems in terms of the client's performance in carrying out an activity, the importance of the activity to the client, and the client's satisfaction with their performance. It has been used successfully in rehabilitation settings (Bodiam, 1999), but limitations to its use have been identified in an acute setting (Ward et al., 1996) and in palliative care (Norris, 1999).

WESTCOTES INDIVIDUALISED OUTCOME MEASURE (WIOM)

The Westcotes Individualised Outcome Measure (WIOM) uses goal-setting to measure outcomes with a scoring system that is able to identify statistically significant change. It provides a formalized system for the method of goal setting.

GOAL SETTING

One of the major problems in using outcome measures routinely in clinical practice is that it might be seen by clinicians to add more work to an already pressured caseload. A system that mirrors routine clinical practice, such as goal setting, can be a way around this. In addition, goal setting has value in palliative care where assessment often needs to be as unobtrusive and low-key as possible. It has a wider application than occupational therapy: it has been shown to work successfully to set multiprofessional goals in a hospice in-patient unit (Needham and Newbury, 2004).

Goal setting is a way of measuring outcomes that involves identifying, in collaboration with patients, realistic, practical, achievable goals relating to a patient's occupational performance. Patients and their families are encouraged to set their own goals based on their present needs and future aspirations. The occupational therapist carries out an assessment to observe the activities that have been identified as problematic. This will give a baseline level of performance, from which change can be measured following occupational therapy intervention. It is an informal method, and as such may lack credibility in formal research, but it has value in day-to-day clinical work as a method that is flexible, adaptable, unobtrusive and client-centred.

A step-by-step guide to setting measurable occupational therapy goals follows. There are four elements to setting client-centred, measurable goals. These are:

- good assessment skills;
- an ability to establish patient/family/carer priorities;
- an understanding of the difference between a goal and an intervention plan;
- skill and confidence in combining patients' stated priorities with the occupational therapy interventions on offer.

ASSESSMENT

The aim of the assessment is to establish a baseline level of performance for the patient. The point from which one is starting needs to be documented clearly. It is this statement of a patient's baseline performance that will be used to measure the outcome of the intervention.

ESTABLISHING PRIORITIES

During the assessment, the occupational therapist will need to establish the patient's/carer's priorities. The following questions may be helpful:

- 'What activities have been important to you?'
- 'What activities do you *need* to be able to do?'
- 'What activities do you *want* to be able to do?'

- 'With what activities are you comfortable receiving help?'
- 'What activities do you want to manage on your own?'

A GOAL VERSUS AN INTERVENTION PLAN

Goals should reflect the following:

- What does the patient want to achieve with regard to occupational performance? For example, Mr Collins will be able to go shopping at his local shops without help, using a motorized wheelchair. Or, Jenny will be able to prepare supper for her children with the aid of a perching stool and a trolley.
- What will the patient know or understand following an occupational therapy intervention? For example, Sylvia will understand the principles of energy conservation, and how to use these in planning her daily activities. Or, Mr and Mrs Young will have a knowledge of the resources offered by their local Independent Living Centre, and understand how to access these if required in the future.

Goals should not reflect what will be done. What will be done forms the intervention plan. 'To carry out a home assessment' is not a goal, it is an intervention plan. Goals will determine the intervention plan, not the other way around.

ADDING IT ALL TOGETHER

At the end of this process, the following data will have been collected:

- a statement of the patient's priority;
- a statement of the patient's baseline performance;
- a statement of the patient's goals;
- an intervention plan.

Here is an example of the process. At all stages, sufficient time needs to be given to patients and carers to enable them to participate fully in the process, and to provide opportunities for the expression of emotion – both positive and negative – relating to the physical, psychological and social consequences of living with illness.

Patient's priority:

- The patient's priority was to be able to sit out in the garden by the fishpond.

Baseline performance:

- Walking ability limited to a distance of 2 yards.
- He was unable to negotiate steps.

Goal:

- Bob would be able to move from his house to his fishpond using a wheelchair propelled by his wife.

Intervention plan:

- Assessment for, and provision of, a wheelchair;
- technician to construct ramp for back door step;
- home visit to ensure that Bob's wife is able to propel the wheelchair easily, with confidence;
- time spent with Bob and his wife.

SUMMARY

A measure of outcome in palliative care needs to reflect the breadth and depth of the occupational therapy process. It must allow for a client-centred approach, with clients identifying those aspects of occupational performance that are important to them. It should take into account the needs of family and carers. It must be flexible and responsive to rapid changes in physical symptoms and emotional outlook.

Occupational therapists should emphasize their wider role in enhancing and enabling occupational performance, and should resist having their contribution measured solely in terms of a patient's independence in activities of daily living. The trend in outcome measurement in occupational therapy is towards client-centred measures of occupational performance, which capture the importance of occupation to health and well-being.

Occupational therapists working with patients or clients with life-limiting illness have to manage the contrast between enhancing the value and meaning of a person's remaining life while simultaneously supporting approaching death.

REFERENCES

Aspinal, F., Addington-Hall, J., Hughes, R. and Higginson, I. J. (2003) Using satisfaction to measure the quality of palliative care: A review of the literature. *Journal of Advanced Nursing*, **42**(4), 324–39.

Bodiam, C. (1999) The use of the Canadian Occupational Performance Measure for the assessment of outcome on a neurorehabilitation unit. *British Journal of Occupational Therapy*, **62**(3), 123–6.

Bye, R. (1998) When clients are dying: Occupational therapists' perspectives. *Occupational Therapy Journal of Research*, **18**(1), 3–24.

Canadian Association of Occupational Therapists (1997) *Enabling Occupation: An occupational therapy perspective*, CAOT Publications, Ottawa.

Department of Health (2000) *The NHS Cancer Plan: A plan for investment, a plan for reform*, HMSO, London.

Eva, G. (2001) *Occupational Therapy Outcomes: Perspectives of patients with advanced cancer*, Unpublished MSc thesis, Oxford Brookes University.

Grahame-Smith, D. (1995) Evidence-based medicine: Socratic dissent. *British Medical Journal*, **310**(6987), 1126–7.

Hasselkus, B. R. (1993) Death in very old age: A personal journey of caregiving. *American Journal of Occupational Therapy*, **47**(8), 717–23.

HOPE (1999) *Survey of the Knowledge and Use of Outcome Measures by HOPE Members*. Unpublished report, College of Occupational Therapists' Specialist Section in HIV/AIDS, Oncology, Palliative Care and Education.

Law, M., Baptiste, S., Carswell, A., McColl, M. A., Polatajko, H. and Pollock, N. (1994) *Canadian Occupational Performance Measure*, 2nd edn, CAOT Publications, Toronto.

Lloyd, C. and Coggles, L. (1990) Psychosocial issues for people with cancer and their families. *Canadian Journal of Occupational Therapy*, **57**(4), 211–15.

Long, A. and Harrison, S. (1996) The balance of evidence. *Health Services Journal* (Health Management Guide), 1–2.

NCHSPCS (1999) *Commissioning Palliative Care Services for the Year 2000*, National Council for Hospice and Specialist Palliative Care Services, London.

Needham, P. R. and Newbury, J. (2004) Goal setting as a measure of outcome in palliative care. *Palliative Medicine*, **18**(5), 444–51.

NICE (2004) *Improving Supportive and Palliative Care for Adults with Cancer: The manual*, National Institute for Clinical Excellence, London.

Norris, A. (1999) A pilot study of an outcome measure in palliative care. *International Journal of Palliative Nursing*, **5**(1), 40–5.

Ward, G., Jagger, C. and Harper, W. M. H. (1996) The Canadian Occupational Performance Measure: What do users consider important? *British Journal of Therapy and Rehabilitation*, **3**(8), 442–52.

RECOMMENDED READING

Assessment of Motor and Process Skills (AMPS) http://www.ampsintl.com/ (accessed on 14/02/2005).

Canadian Occupational Performance Measure http://www.caot.ca/copm/ (accessed on 14/02/05).

Clarke, C., Sealey-Lapes, C. and Kotsch, L. (2001) *Outcome Measures Information Pack for Occupational Therapy*, College of Occupational Therapists, London.

Functional Independence Measure (FIM) http://www.udsmr.org/ (accessed on 14/02/2005).

Palliative care Outcomes Scale (POS) http://www.kcl.ac.uk/depsta/palliative/pos/index.html (accessed on 14/02/05).

Schedule for the Evaluation of Individualised Quality of Life (SEIQoL) and Schedule for the Evaluation of Individualised Quality of Life – Direct Weighting (SEIQoL-DW), Department of Psychology, Royal College of Surgeons in Ireland Medical School, 123 St Stephen's Green, Dublin 2, Ireland.

Westcotes Individualised Outcome Measure (WIOM) Occupational Therapy Department, Westcotes Health Centre, Fosse Road South, Leicester LE3 0LP.

Appendix 1

ADVICE ON EXPLORING HOW TO WORK WITH PEOPLE WHO ARE POTENTIALLY DYING AND MORE SPECIFICALLY THE BEREAVEMENT

- Be aware of your own feelings. When showing empathy, it is appropriate to be sad or angry at what can be a desperately sad situation. But you do have to keep yourself healthy and deal with your own feelings too.
- You can't solve everyone's problems. That's not what you are there for; recognize your own limitations and inadequacies in some issues. You are not expected to have all the answers. Don't try too hard.
- Be in touch with your own parenting instincts. You will want to make the pain go away, to make it better by your living and caring, but you can't!
- Not all questions have answers. Life and death are a mystery and perhaps helping the bereaved to ask the right questions can be your gift to them.
- Don't ignore the death. It has happened, and pretending otherwise only puts off dealing with it.
- Be practical and share your time. One helpful action is worth a thousand clever words, a little time may be all that is needed.
- Be ready to listen. Allow the bereaved time and space to tell their story and express their anger.
- Remember the uniqueness of grief. Every person has the right to react in his or her own way.
- Remember that grieving takes time and you cannot rush adapting to change.
- Coax, but don't bully. Remember the thin dividing line between the two.
- Urge patience, and be careful to watch the platitudes.
- Be alert and notice signs of deterioration and improvement.
- Don't slink away. Everyone else will.
- Remember that professional help may be needed in the end.

Rev. Tom Gordon (1995) in Cooper (1997)

Occupational Therapy in Oncology and Palliative Care. Edited by J. Cooper
© 2006 John Wiley & Sons Ltd

Appendix 2

FACTORS INFLUENCING WHETHER OR NOT STAFF COPE WHEN WORKING IN POTENTIALLY STRESSFUL SITUATIONS

- personal awareness of the job;
- maintaining a healthy balance between work and social life;
- preparedness for the job being carried out;
- organizational issues relating to management and ensuring support is given to staff;
- availability of this support. If not available, this increases stress;
- willingness to accept and make use of this support;
- ability to control working hours. Aspects of the job including notewriting should be integral to working hours – work as well as time-owing should not be allowed to accumulate;
- taking a break when it is needed;
- ability to devise one's own personal stress-management strategies, including recognizing when one is becoming tired and snappy and looking at what is going wrong.

Faulkner and Maguire (1994)

Occupational Therapy in Oncology and Palliative Care. Edited by J. Cooper
© 2006 John Wiley & Sons Ltd

Appendix 3

RECOMMENDATIONS FOR COMMUNICATION IN INTERVIEWS

DO

Allow time
Ensure privacy
Respect confidentiality
Let the patient talk
Listen to what the patient says
Be sensitive to non-verbal cues such as facial expression
Gauge the need for information on an individual basis
Permit painful topics to be discussed
Permit silences
Very selectively use humour only when absolutely certain of its appropriateness

DON'T

Assume you know what is troubling the person
Give false reassurance
Overload the client with information
Feel obliged to keep talking all the time
Withhold information
Tell lies
Criticize or make judgements
Give direct advice about psychological matters

Brewin (1991) in Cooper (1997)

Occupational Therapy in Oncology and Palliative Care. Edited by J. Cooper
© 2006 John Wiley & Sons Ltd

Appendix 4

PROACTIVE PRINCIPLES WHEN DEALING WITH HOSTILITY

- Recognize early warning signs
- Use reason and be reasonable
- Relate
- Reply to the underlying emotion
- Retreat – this is entirely appropriate and permissible
- Respond and react
- Report
- Record
- Review and re-examine.

Lanciotti and Hopkins (1995)

Occupational Therapy in Oncology and Palliative Care. Edited by J. Cooper
© 2006 John Wiley & Sons Ltd

Appendix 5

THE THERAPEUTIC EFFECTS OF FACILITATING SELF-EXPRESSION

- it increases self-esteem by allowing clients to reflect on what they have achieved;
- it enables clients to emphasize their individuality at a time when they may be losing their own identity due to frequent hospital appointments, hospital admissions and gradual institutionalization;
- it strengthens their identity as productive individuals;
- it gives them the opportunity to share life experiences with others so helping them see the client in their former life roles;
- it enables them to accept the stage of life at which they find themselves;
- it encourages them to air their concerns;
- it helps the problem-solving process by enabling others to identify the specific problems;
- it allows the occupational therapist to help the client to turn negative thoughts into positive thoughts;
- it helps clients provide meaning, a sense of fulfillment and purpose to their lives.

Stoter (1996) in Cooper (1997)

Occupational Therapy in Oncology and Palliative Care. Edited by J. Cooper
© 2006 John Wiley & Sons Ltd

Appendix 6

ANXIETY MANAGEMENT ASSESSMENT

NAME

❑ What makes me feel anxious?

❑ What physical symptoms do I usually experience when I feel anxious?

❑ What thoughts do I have during times when I feel anxious?

❑ What do I do when I feel anxious?

❑ What activities do I find difficult when I feel anxious?

Occupational Therapy in Oncology and Palliative Care. Edited by J. Cooper
© 2006 John Wiley & Sons Ltd

Appendix 7

A PERSONAL PLAN TO HELP MANAGE ANXIETY

NAME

Breathing techniques:

Relaxation techniques:

Some useful positive phrases to use if I'm feeling anxious:

- When preparing for an activity:

- During an activity:

- And after an activity . . . praising myself!

Small goals to help me achieve tasks that sometimes make me feel anxious:

Appendix 8

SIMPLE BREATHING TECHNIQUE

INSTRUCTIONS

1. Loosen any tight clothing, position yourself comfortably either lying or sitting, but ensuring that your back is supported.
2. Close your eyes if you wish.
3. Keep your shoulders and upper chest relaxed.
4. Place your hand flat on your stomach.
5. Inhale slowly (through your nose if possible).
   As you breathe in, your stomach should gently swell underneath your hand (this should not be a forced movement using your abdominal muscles).
6. Remember to keep your shoulders and upper chest relaxed.
7. Exhale slowly through your mouth.
8. Your stomach will gently flatten beneath your hand.
9. Pause, then repeat steps 2–9.

During the exercise, think of a positive word or phrase, such as 'I am relaxed' or 'I feel calm'.

Appendix 9

CHALLENGING NEGATIVE THINKING

NAME

What are my thoughts when I am feeling anxious?	Are these thoughts reasonable? If not, why not?	How can I consider these thoughts in a more positive way?

Occupational Therapy in Oncology and Palliative Care. Edited by J. Cooper
© 2006 John Wiley & Sons Ltd

Appendix 10

OCCUPATIONAL THERAPY DEPARTMENT

RELAXATION PROGRAMME ASSESSMENT

Name: Hospital No.:

Do you have any previous experience of relaxation?

How does anxiety effect you?

Symptoms: Physical   Thoughts   Emotions

What are your expectations of relaxation?

Occupational Therapy in Oncology and Palliative Care. Edited by J. Cooper
© 2006 John Wiley & Sons Ltd

OT: Date:

OUTCOME   Date:

COMMENTS

Session 1

Session 2

Session 3

Session 4

Appendix 11

RELAXATION FEEDBACK FORM

NAME ....

Rate how tense/relaxed you feel a scale of 0–10, both before and after the relaxation session

SCALE: 0 = VERY RELAXED
          10 = VERY TENSE

DATE	BEFORE/AFTER	LOW	TENSION	HIGH
		0 ———————————————— 10		

1.

2.

3.

4.

Appendix 12

RELAXATION: RELEASE-ONLY TECHNIQUE

INSTRUCTIONS FOR CARRYING OUT THIS TECHNIQUE

- It is important that before beginning this technique you are comfortable with the progressive muscle relaxation technique.
- The 'Release-only' technique focuses on relaxing muscles in order to achieve full body relaxation.
- It depends upon your ability to recognize the difference between clenched muscles and relaxed ones.
- This is a technique that, once it has been practised, can be used in most situations (even in public places/in social situations) to relieve stress/tension and achieve relaxation.

A. First make yourself completely comfortable. Allow your body to sink into the chair or floor // let your feet and legs gently roll outwards // enjoy the feeling of resting . . . of being completely supported.

B. Now become aware of your breathing // Follow the breath as it comes into and goes out of your body // Don't try to control it in any way – just observe the natural rhythm of your breathing.
As you breathe out, imagine your whole body deflating, growing limp and heavy.
Each time you breathe out, imagine that you are letting tension flow out of your body and mind // Focus on the word 'calm' as the breath flows gently in and out of your body.

C. Now relax your forehead // smoothing out all the lines // Keep breathing deeply . . . and now relax your eyebrows // Just let all the tension melt away, all the way down to your jaw // Let it all go // Now let your lips separate and relax your tongue // Breathe in and out and relax your throat // Notice how peaceful and loose your entire face feels now //.

D. Roll your head gently and feel your neck relax // Release your shoulders. Just let them drop all the way down // Your neck is loose, and your shoulders are heavy and low // Now let the relaxation travel down through your arms to your fingertips // Your arms are heavy and loose // Your lips are still separated because your jaw is relaxed, too //.

E. Breathe in deeply and feel your stomach expand and then your chest // Hold your breath for a moment* // then breathe out slowly, in a smooth stream through your mouth //.

F. Let the feeling of relaxation spread to your stomach // Feel all the muscles in your abdomen release their tension, as it assumes its natural shape // Relax your waist and relax your back // Continue to breathe deeply // Notice how loose and heavy the upper half of your body feels //.

G. And now relax the lower half of your body // Feel your buttocks sink into the chair // Relax your thighs // Relax your knees // Feel the relaxation travel through your calves to your ankles // to the bottoms of your feet, all the way down to the tips of your toes // Your feet feel warm and heavy on the floor/bed in front of you // With each breath, feel the relaxation deepen //.

H. Now scan your body for tension as you continue to breathe // Your legs are relaxed // Your back is relaxed // Your shoulders and arms are relaxed // Your face is relaxed // There's only a feeling of peace and warmth and relaxation //.

I. If any muscle felt hard to relax, turn your attention to it now // Is it your back? // Your shoulders? // Your thighs? // Your jaw? // Tune in to the muscle and now tense it // Hold it tighter and release // Feel it join the rest of your body in a deep, deep relaxation //.

J. Now bring your attention back to your breathing // Feel your stomach and chest rise and fall slowly as you breathe in . . . and . . . out // Take a moment to listen to the music and appreciate this feeling of relaxation. **(Longer pause)**

K. Slowly start to focus back on the room in which you are in // Still breathing in a calm, steady manner // When you are ready, open your eyes // Remember to have a stretch // and very gradually bring yourself back into a sitting position //.

---

* Not to use with breathless patients

Appendix 13

GUIDED VISUALIZATION – 'COTTAGE BY THE SEA'

Instructions:

- If using this exercise on its own, take participants through the following short general relaxation instructions at the beginning.

1. First make yourself completely comfortable // Allow your body to sink into the floor // Let your legs and feet flop outwards // If you are lying on the floor, have your arms resting on the floor beside you // Enjoy the feeling of resting, of being completely supported // let your eyes close // Make sure that your jaw is loose and that your teeth are not clenched together // Ensure your tongue is lying gently in the bottom of your mouth // Have a slight gap between your upper and lower teeth and let your lips be slightly parted.

2. Now become aware of your breathing // Follow the breath as it comes into and goes out of your body // Do not try to control it in any way // Just observe the natural rhythm of your breathing // As you breathe out, imagine your whole body deflating, growing limp and heavy // Each time you breathe out, imagine that you are letting tension flow out of your body and mind //.

3. Now that your body is relaxed, take yourself in your imagination to the garden of a cottage by the sea // You are sitting in a comfortable garden chair with plump cushions // All around you are the flowers of the cottage garden and you have a wonderful view out to the sea // You sit in the warmth of the sun, listening to the lazy drone of insects and the sound of the gulls crying overhead // In the distance you hear the rhythmic beating of the waves on the beach below //.

4. After a while, you get up from your chair and walk across the brilliant, sun-warmed grass of the lawn // You make your way down a flight of steps that leads directly onto the wide, smooth, sandy beach // You are quite alone on your stretch of sand, although you can see tiny figures playing in the distance and hear a faint sound of their voices from far

Occupational Therapy in Oncology and Palliative Care. Edited by J. Cooper
© 2006 John Wiley & Sons Ltd

away // You take off your shoes, and walk over the pale, warm, dry sand down towards the water's edge // Feel the warmth coming from the sand beneath your feet, feel the sand between your toes //.

5. As you get nearer to the sea, the sand becomes smooth, hard and damp // Feel this new texture, the sand is perfectly smooth, with only here and there a tiny pink shell glinting in the light of the sun // Now you can come to the water's edge // You watch the sparkling foam running up the beach towards you, and you let the warm, shallow water flow around your ankles // You look out to sea, and notice a sail on the horizon // You follow it with your eyes as it moves round the headland and out of sight // Then you walk along the water's edge, enjoying the rhythmic swish of the waves swirling around your ankles, the sunlight dancing on the water //.

6. Now you turn back towards the cottage // You walk back over the smooth, hard sand // Over the pale, powdery sand // You go up the steps which lead back on to the lawn // The grass feels cool and refreshing to your warm bare sandy feet // You sit down in your chair again, allow your eyes to close and bask in the warmth of the late afternoon sun //.

// Long Pause //

7. Begin to concentrate once again on your breathing // Imagine the tension leaving your body with every breath out and relaxation entering with every breath in // Start to bring yourself slowly back to the room where we are // In your own time open your eyes //.

Appendix 14

CASE STUDIES

CASE STUDY 1 – REFLECTIVE CASE HISTORY

Mrs D

Age: 48

Diagnosis: Metastatic breast cancer

MEDICAL HISTORY

Diagnosis of breast cancer was made five years ago and Mrs D had a right mastectomy and adjuvant chemotherapy and radiotherapy. Last year, diagnosis was made of metastases spread to anterior mediasternum, lung and kidneys. Mrs D had also developed mild lymphoedema of her right arm. This year, Mrs D was admitted with weakness in both her legs and there was a query of spinal cord compression. After diagnostic scans, metastatic spread to the meninges was discovered. She was treated with radiotherapy, steroids and chemotherapy.

Mrs D also had insulin controlled diabetes, which meant that the patient was often admitted for her chemotherapy to monitor her diabetes following chemotherapy.

SOCIAL HISTORY

Married, with two children; a 16-year-old daughter and a 12-year-old son. She was working as a teacher with learning disability children.

Occupational Therapy in Oncology and Palliative Care. Edited by J. Cooper
© 2006 John Wiley & Sons Ltd

OCCUPATIONAL THERAPY INTERVENTION

At initial diagnosis Mrs D was referred to the breast support group. She was introduced to the following programme of education about cancer and its treatments. She was taught cognitive behavioural techniques to help manage negative thinking, and her emotions. The occupational therapy was involved in introducing managing stress and teaching of relaxation techniques. After this seven week course there was no further occupational therapy input.

When re-admitted last year with kidney, anterior mediasternum and lung metastases she was referred to occupational therapy for breathlessness management. Her social situation had changed, she was now divorced and was in a bitter battle with her husband to move out of their home. Her parents bought her and the children their own home. Mrs D planned to start a new job in January working in administration part time.

Occupational therapy intervention:

- assess how shortness of breath affects activity, i.e. activity of daily living tasks and transfer skills;
- advise on anxiety management, breath control and previously learned relaxation exercises;
- provide equipment if needed (at this stage Mrs D refused to consider any equipment at home, feeling she had a young son at home and did not want the home to look like a hospital. She did, however, ask to be referred to her local social services for consideration of a downstairs toilet);
- advise on lifestyle management and activity scheduling.

She was re-admitted this year with laptomeningeal swelling of the brain, and is now unable to walk. The medical team hope that following radiotherapy, steroids and chemotherapy her condition may improve. With her parents' help she is building a downstairs toilet and shower cubicle. Her daughter is now in university and her son is taking his school examinations.

OCCUPATIONAL THERAPY INTERVENTION

- discussion with Mrs D on environmental assessment and adaptations to suit her needs. Following radiotherapy to the brain it was clear that Mrs D would not regain the use of her legs to walk. Discussion took place with Mrs D and her father about the building works taking place, which needed to be adequate for wheelchair

access. Agreed for occupational therapy and community occupational therapy to meet with builders to ensure there would be adequate space for wheelchair access to the toilet and shower and to consider what type of shower adaptations would be needed to be provided by the builder;
- provide a wheelchair;
- assess and provide advice on manual handling, transfers and mobility;
- regular review to take into account fluctuations in her condition and to help Mrs D, her children and her parents cope with deterioration. Discussions were carried out with Mrs D about being referred to the family support worker, particularly as her son was not coping with her deterioration;
- assess Mrs D's cognition.

THE AIM OF THE ABOVE OCCUPATIONAL THERAPY INTERVENTION IS AS FOLLOWS

- maintain Mrs D at home for as long as possible;
- maximize her independence with personal care tasks;
- maintain her safety at home;
- provide support for the family particularly if their condition is deteriorating.

REFLECTIONS ON THE CARE OF MRS D PROVIDED BY OCCUPATIONAL THERAPY

In her last admission this year, the occupational therapy became very involved with Mrs D, a very determined person, who fiercely fought to be independent. What surprised the occupational therapy was how rapidly she deteriorated, and despite working very closely with her builders and local occupational therapy services we were unable to get Mrs D home. The occupational therapy was also unable to provide family support for her son and her parents. It is hoped that the family would be supported via the school pastoral support services. An alternative approach would have been to discuss the need for family support earlier with Mrs D. The rapid and unusual development of her disease made it difficult to reflect on any changes in occupational therapy practice.

CASE STUDY 2 – PAEDIATRIC CASE STUDY

Steven

Age: 15

Diagnosis: Duchenne muscular dystrophy

Steven attends a mainstream school. Before he began at his secondary school his community paediatric occupational therapist, Lynn, assessed and provided advice and recommendations to the school to help him access the school environment and curriculum. She has been working with Steven for several years and has seen him lose his motor skills over time. She assessed for Steven's first wheelchair and reviews his seating needs regularly. She has advised the school on computer use for all of his work, and has provided support and advice to teachers and care assistants on inclusion in all activities, as well as explaining moving and handling procedures, e.g. when using the toilet at school. Lynn liaises with the social services occupational therapist in the home about a hoist, bathing equipment and wheelchair access. Lynn is aware of the stages of Duchenne muscular dystrophy and is sensitive to Steven's need for independence in his teens as he becomes physically more dependent. Lynn knows Steven's family well now.

Steven has occasional stays at a children's hospice for respite and an opportunity to meet other teenagers with Duchenne muscular dystrophy. He knows the staff, including the occupational therapist. At 17, Steven contracts pneumonia and his condition deteriorates. He is transferred from the hospital to the hospice for terminal stage care. The palliative care occupational therapist works with the care team to make Steven comfortable, through positioning and a moving and handling assessment including equipment needed, e.g. for bathing. She spends some time with Steven who is showing signs of anxiety, which affects his breathing. She shares a relaxation technique with Steven using imagery to help calm him. The occupational therapist is aware of the anxiety of the parents and as part of the hospice team she spends time listening to, and talking with, them. Steven's younger sister is noticeably withdrawn. The occupational therapist involves her with the relaxation for her brother, and talks with her about her understanding of her brother's condition.

This occupational therapist is in contact with Lynn and keeps her informed. Lynn visits Steven and his parents at the hospice. Steven dies at the hospice. The hospice occupational therapist is involved as part of the care team in the care of Steven's body after he dies and works with the family in bereavement support for some time afterwards. The occupational therapist regularly sees Steven's sister at the sibling bereavement group.

CASE STUDY 3 – CREATIVITY

Woman

Age: 42

Diagnosis: Cerebral metastases

The patient has rapidly progressing communication problems due to cerebral metastases and finds that her inability to have a conversation with her husband is further adding to friction within the relationship. They had always shared everything and now she was unable to recount the activities that she had been involved in, limiting their conversation considerably. By using a small ring file as a diary, in which the staff could write, and by including digital photographs of the patient involved in her activities, the husband could use this information to initiate a discourse between them, and to ask closed questions. It also facilitated a situation in which information could be relayed to the day hospice staff so that any issues that could be dealt with by them could be discussed with the patient and not her husband – returning control and therefore self-esteem to the patient.

As well as providing an overview of the patient's activities, using the diary provided the opportunity:

- to emphasize positive achievements and provide a record;
- to suggest alternative ways to optimize function, which could be followed up at home;
- to motivate the patient and carer;
- to address certain relationship issues;
- for self-expression and catharsis;
- to leave behind memories in the form of the diary pages themselves, photographs, poems, letters and a written record of the interactions of the individuals concerned.

CASE STUDY 4 – CREATIVITY

Joan

Age: 60

Diagnosis: Advanced lung cancer

Joan's pleasures in life revolved around entertaining. She had always been the one in the family who organized and prepared the parties and every Christmas family and friends gathered at her home for a feast of homemade goodies. This Christmas, however, it was clear that she would not be able to fulfil that role as before. She was distraught at the thought that she would be letting the family down and that someone else would be taking over her role. Her daughters were only too happy to do the cooking and the other preparations but Joan knew that they had never catered for a large number of people and worried about how they would cope. We started to make a list together of what had to be done and soon Joan had identified tasks for the various members of the family and friends to help. She made the crackers in the activity group and put small gifts inside – some that she had made herself, some she had bought and others that were pieces of her own jewellery that she wanted to give to her granddaughters. The family asked her advice about the different aspects of the day and everything was carried out as Joan wished. In this way she could feel satisfied that she had made her own contribution to what by all accounts was a very successful day.

Appendix 15

MANAGING YOUR DAILY ACTIVITIES AND COPING WITH BREATHLESSNESS

REMEMBER THE 5 'P's

PRIORITIZE

Consider which activities are important to you each day, and prioritize those activities for which you would like to conserve your energy.

Try to cut out unnecessary tasks in order to conserve your energy.

PLAN

Organize your activities as effectively as possible in order to conserve as much energy as you can.

Consider which times of the day are best for you to be active or at rest.

Try not to do too much in any one day, and plan your activities for the week ahead as much as possible.

PACE

It is important to balance periods of activity with periods of rest. You may need to rest during an activity and allow yourself a little extra time to get things done.

POSITION

Work out a position that is comfortable for you when you feel breathless and practise this so that you can help yourself.

Occupational Therapy in Oncology and Palliative Care. Edited by J. Cooper
© 2006 John Wiley & Sons Ltd

Think about your posture and try to maintain this so that you avoid becoming uncomfortable and conserve your energy.

PERMISSION

Give yourself permission NOT to do activities which result in your becoming breathless and tired.

Instead of thinking along the lines of 'I must', 'I ought', try and change the way you think about things and say to yourself 'I choose to do . . .' 'I wish to do . . .' instead.

Ewer-Smith et al. (2002)

Appendix 16

A PERSONAL PLAN TO HELP YOU REGAIN CONTROL WHEN BREATHLESS

NAME: HOSPITAL NO.

Position

Methods which relax shoulders and upper chest

Techniques which assist in gentle, lower chest breathing

Techniques to regain control

Relaxation techniques

Occupational Therapy in Oncology and Palliative Care. Edited by J. Cooper
© 2006 John Wiley & Sons Ltd

Practise the following techniques . . .

Ewer-Smith *et al.* (2002)

Appendix 17

TOP TIPS!

- ❑ Take your time when walking; take frequent rests if you need to, especially when walking up gentle slopes. Check if your local shopping centre has wheelchairs to borrow, if necessary.
- ❑ Avoid using the stairs too many times in any one day. If possible, use them once in the morning and once in the evening. (This is where planning comes in!)
- ❑ Avoid bending down where possible; sit down when emptying the washing machine, place items on a table when organizing them, use a Helping Hand.
- ❑ Sit down as much as possible when washing and dressing, and avoid bending as much as possible. Have a seat while you dry yourself after a bath or shower.
- ❑ Inform friends that you may take a little more time to answer the phone; make sure that you sit while talking.

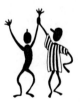

Ewer-Smith *et al.* (2002)

Occupational Therapy in Oncology and Palliative Care. Edited by J. Cooper
© 2006 John Wiley & Sons Ltd

REFERENCES

Brewin, T. B. (1997) Dilemmas faced by occupational therapists. *Occupational Therapy in Oncology and Palliative Care* (ed. J. Cooper), Whurr, London, p. 19.

Ewer-Smith, C., Patterson, S., Lowrie, D., Vockins, H. and Watterson, J. (2002) *Relaxation Programme*, The Royal Marsden Hospital Occupational Therapy Department. Unpublished.

Faulkner, A. and Maguire, P. (1994) Dilemmas faced by occupational therapists. *Occupational Therapy in Oncology and Palliative Care* (ed. J. Cooper), Whurr, London, p. 15.

Gordon, Rev. T. (1997) Dilemmas faced by occupational therapists. *Occupational Therapy in Oncology and Palliative Care* (ed. J. Cooper), Whurr, London, p. 14.

Lanciotti, L. and Hopkins, A. (1995) Dilemmas faced by occupational therapists. *Occupational Therapy in Oncology and Palliative Care* (ed. J. Cooper), Whurr, London, p. 21.

Stoter, D. (1997) Dilemmas faced by occupational therapists. *Occupational Therapy in Oncology and Palliative Care* (ed. J. Cooper), Whurr, London, pp. 27–8.

Glossary

Adenocarcinomas arise from the cells of tissues in which glandular structures are common features, for example, the thyroid gland, stomach or pancreas.

Aesthesia is perception, feeling or sensation.

AIDS is the diagnosis of acquired immune deficiency syndrome in which an individual's CD4 count falls below 200 and where there have been diagnosed one or more from a standard list of opportunistic infections.

ALL (acute lymphoblastic leukaemia) accounts for over 25% of childhood cancers in Britain and requires drugs less powerful or severe than for AML. It usually responds quickly to drugs that do not damage the marrow as seriously as those for AML (see AML).

Allogenic transplantation involves cells that are transplanted from the donor into the recipient from the same species, i.e. human to human, as opposed to animal to human.

Alveolar pertains to the minute divisions of glands and air sacs of the lungs.

AML (acute myeloblastic leukaemia) is a type of leukaemia requiring very intensive chemotherapy that completely kills the whole of the bone marrow, including the normal elements, with the hope and intention that the normal marrow will regenerate without the cancerous blood cells reappearing.

Anaplasia is a characteristic of tumour tissue where there is loss of differentiation of cells and their orientation to one another.

Ankylosing spondylitis is a rheumatoid arthritis affecting the spine, characterized by painful stiffening of joints and ligaments.

Anorexia is the uncontrolled lack or loss of appetite for food, usually due to nausea, caused by symptoms of the disease or treatment, e.g. radiotherapy and/or chemotherapy.

Antiretroviral therapy uses a therapeutic drug that stops or suppresses the activity of a retrovirus such as HIV.

Anxiolytics are medications used to reduce anxiety, tension or agitation.

Aphasia is the inability to word find or perform the coordinated tasks required for speech.

Apraxia is the inability to execute a skilled or learned motor skill, not related to paralysis or lack of comprehension, caused by a cortical lesion.

Occupational Therapy in Oncology and Palliative Care. Edited by J. Cooper
© 2006 John Wiley & Sons Ltd

Arthralgia is pain in the joints.

Astrocytoma is the commonest of brain tumours, arising from astrocyte cells in the brain.

Ataxia is the loss of irregularity of muscular coordination and action due to neurological impairment, though the power necessary to make movements is still present.

Attention is the ability to focus, shift and divide attention between different tasks.

Autologous transplantation involves cells that are transplanted into the recipient from the person's own marrow following chemotherapy.

Batten disease is a congenital disorder occurring between the ages of 5 and 10, causing the child to suddenly go blind, suffer from seizures and mental deterioration, usually resulting in death before the age of 20.

Body cavity effusions are areas of excess fluid that flow into a body cavity, e.g. the abdomen. The fluid is produced in the body in response to illness and needs to escape from the body tissues where it causes damage so the body flushes it into a cavity.

Bronchi (sing.: **bronchus**) are the tubes into which the windpipe divides, one going to either lung. It also applies to the divisions of these tubes distributed throughout the lungs, the smallest being bronchioles.

Bronchiectasis is persistent and progressive dilation of bronchi and bronchioles due to inflammation from lung infection, obstruction due to tumour or congenital respiratory disease.

Burkitt's lymphoma is a form of malignant lymphoma usually found in central Africa, with abdominal tumour.

Cachexia is a marked state of malnutrition and general ill health.

Candida is a fungus affecting moist areas of the body, e.g. thrush in the mouth or genital areas.

Carcinoma is a malignant tumour originating from an organ with a surface, either an external surface such as the skin, or an internal surface such as the lining of the bronchial airways or gastrointestinal tract.

Carpal tunnel syndrome presents as a complex of symptoms resulting from compression of the median nerve in the carpal tunnel, with pain and burning or tingling paraesthesias in the fingers and hand, up to the elbow.

Castleman's Syndrome has solitary masses of tissues of the lymphatic system occurring in mediastinum (chest space between the lungs).

CCD is the Centre for Communicable Diseases.

Cerebral toxoplasmosis is an acute or chronic, widespread disease affecting the brain, transmitted by direct exposure to the source of infection in body fluids.

CML (chronic myeloid leukaemia) develops in an older age group, treated by alpha-interferon orally, which is much gentler than treatment for **AML**.

Cognition involves the ability of the mind to perceive, think and remember.

Cortico-steroids is the generic term for the group of hormones with a cortisone-like action. They reduce inflammation that may result from radiotherapy or from infections.

Cryptococcal meningitis is an opportunistic infection caused by fungus and involves the membranes surrounding the brain and spinal cord, which may lead to severe headache, confusion, sensitivity to light, blurred vision, fever and speech difficulties.

CT scan (computed tomography scan) demonstrates the distortion or enlargement of an organ or a change in density and thus shows the extent of infiltration of primary tumours and delineates metastatic spread to adjacent lymph nodes and other structures.

CVA is a cerebrovascular accident or stroke.

Cytomegalovirus infections are characterized by enlarged cells particularly in the lungs in adults and salivary glands in children.

Cytotoxic drugs enter the bloodstream and destroy cancer cells by interfering with the cells' ability to grow and divide. Although normal cells can be damaged, most healthy tissue grows back again.

Dementia is an organic mental disorder characterized by loss of intellectual abilities.

Demyelination is loss, removal or destruction of the myelin sheath surrounding nerves.

Denervation is resection or removal of the nerves to an organ or part.

Duchenne muscular dystrophy is a specific form of muscular dystrophy that is inherited as a sex-linked recessive trait, confined to young males. There is degeneration and death of skeletal muscle fibres, which are replaced by fat and fibrous tissue, resulting in muscle weakness. Advance cases include respiratory muscle weakness.

Dysfunction is difficulty in normal action, disturbance or impairment in the functioning of an organ.

Dysphagia is difficulty in swallowing.

Dysphasia refers to impairment in speech due to the difficulties in coordination and word finding.

Dyspnoea is difficult or laboured breathing.

Dyspraxia is partial inability to perform coordinated acts, for example, dressing dyspraxia might involve difficulty in recognizing body parts and clothing.

Edwards syndrome is a congenital disorder caused by a baby having an extra copy of chromosome 18 (three instead of two), a large number of different malformed organs and malformed physical features of the face and skeleton. In most cases the baby dies before it is born; 90% of babies born alive die within a year of birth.

Encephalopathy is any degenerative disease of the brain.

Endothelium is the membrane lining various vessels and cavities of the body, such as lungs, blood vessels, heart, abdominal cavity and joints. It consists of a fibrous layer covered with thin flat cells that form a perfectly a perfectly smooth surface and that secrete fluid for its lubrication.

Epidermolysis bullosa is a group of rare inherited disorders in which blistering of the skin occurs in response to skin trauma, resulting in internal blistering, malnutrition, infections and loss of function in hands and feet.

Epithelial cancer is a cancer of the cells covering the internal and external surfaces of the body, including the lining of vessels and other small cavities.

Ergonomics is the science that relates individuals to their environment in order to achieve the most efficient use of energy or resources.

Erythropoietic agents are used in drug therapy which stimulates the production of red blood corpuscles (erythrocytes).

Ewing's sarcoma is a highly malignant metastatic tumour of the primitive small round cells of the bone, usually occurring in the diaphyses of long bones, ribs and flat bones of children or adolescents.

Fibrosing alveolitis is a progressive inflammatory condition resulting in diffuse alveolar damage and fibrosis (hardening) of lung tissue.

Granulomatous refers to new growth made up of tissues that grow over any raw surface as the first step in healing of wounds.

Guillain-Barré Syndrome is an acute infective virus resulting in symptoms ranging from peripheral neuropathy (loss of feeling and use in the body's extremities) to temporary loss of movement and sensation in all main nerves and muscle groups resulting in whole body paralysis.

Hemianopia is partial loss of the field of vision, usually affecting a specific quadrant or half of visual field.

Hemiparesis is partial paralysis or weakness affecting one side of the body.

Hemiplegia is paralysis of one side of the body.

Hepatomegaly symptoms arise following enlargement of the liver.

Herpes simplex virus causes blisters on the lips, nostrils and lining of the eyelids.

Histogenesis is the formation or development of tissues from the undifferentiated cells of the germ layer of the embryo.

HIV is a type of retrovirus (human immunodeficiency virus) that induces AIDS (acquired immune deficiency syndrome), which can be fatal.

Hodgkin's disease cells appear under the microscope to be quite different from those of non-Hodgkin's lymphoma. Hodgkin's disease has painless, enlarged lymph nodes that spread in a logical anatomic progression. It peaks at age 30, then again later in life.

Homeostasis is the ability of the body to correct imbalances, e.g. when there is a problem in the body such as high levels of CO_2, the body stabilizes it.

Hyperaesthesia is a disturbance in sensation resulting in increased sensitivity, particularly a painful sensation from a normally painless touch stimulus.

Hypercalcaemia is excess of calcium in the blood resulting in confusion, disorientation, fatigue, muscle weakness, depression, anorexia, nausea and constipation.

Immunosuppression occurs when the body's immune system is suppressed or compromised due to illness or treatment.

Inattention is the inability to be able to focus or shift attention between specific tasks.

Kaposi's sarcoma is a malignant skin tumour seen in PLWHA, occurring on the face, but also within the intestines and lungs.

Leiomyosarcoma is a malignant tumour of smooth muscle origin, e.g. hollow internal organs and walls of blood vessels. It can occur almost anywhere in the body, most commonly in the uterus and gastrointestinal tract.

Lesions originally meant an injury, but are now applied generally to all disease changes in organs and tissues.

Leukaemia is a progressive malignant disease of the blood-forming organs, characterized by distorted proliferation and development of leukocytes and their precursors in the blood and bone marrow.

Leukodystrophy is a type of hereditary disease resulting in neurological problems due to problems with the myelin sheaths of the nerve fibres, poor coordination and deterioration in functional abilities.

Lipoatrophy is loss of subcutaneous fat.

Lipodystrophy is any disturbance of fat metabolism.

Lymphatic system is the collective term for the lymphatic vessels and tissue that carry excess fluid away from the body's tissues to the bloodstream.

Lymphoedema is the accumulation of lymph fluid in the tissues resulting in swelling caused by obstruction of the lymphatic vessels.

Lymphoma is a malignant disorder of the lymphatic system, glands become enlarged during infections, often with night sweats, fever and weight loss.

Lymphoproliferative disorders are characterized by proliferation of lymphoid tissue, affecting the lymphatic system.

Mastectomy is the surgical removal of the breast and breast tissue.

Meninges are the surrounding membranes of the brain and spinal cord.

Metastasize is to spread to another part of the body, usually via blood vessels, lymph channels or spinal fluid.

MRI scan (magnetic resonance imaging scan) is used particularly for spinal cord, brain and sarcoma and evidence of bone metastases. It takes images in any plane and can be repeated more frequently than x-rays, as it does not involve exposure to radiation.

Mucopolysaccharide is a biochemical term for the components of body proteins.

Mycobacterium avium intracellulare is an opportunistic infection of PLWHA, causing respiratory tract infections.

Myeloma is a tumour composed of cells of the type normally found in the bone marrow.

Myocardial cells are those of the heart muscle.

Myopathy is a functional disturbance or pathological change in the muscles.

Neglect is the lack of awareness of a body part or area of the body, usually linked with hemiplegia.

Neoplasm is new abnormal growth of tissue or tumour.

Neoplastic activity refers to new and abnormal growth activity of cells.

Neuroblastoma is a brain tumour of the particular part of the gland that manufactures adrenaline. It is treated by surgery and/or radiation; chemotherapy is used in advanced cases.

Neurones are nerve cells.

Neuropathy is a functional disturbance or pathological change in the peripheral nervous system.

Neutropenia is the reduction in the number of neutrophilic leucocytes per cubic millimetre of circulating blood to a figure below that found in healthy individuals, i.e. low white blood cell count.

Niemann Pick Syndrome is a family of symptoms, whose clinical signs include foam cells in the blood and marrow and neurological degeneration, most commonly presenting in Ashkenazi Jewish children.

Non-Hodgkin's lymphoma (NHL) is a group of lymphomas that differ in important ways from Hodgkin's lymphomas. The term covers a wide spectrum characterized by malignant transformation of lymph nodes.

Oedema is the excessive accumulation of fluid in body tissues.

OIs are opportunistic infections that are allowed to occur in the body in an immunosuppressed state.

Oncogenes are a specific segment of DNA that confers the property of malignancy.

Oncology is the study and practice of treating tumours.

Opioids are synthetic narcotics resembling opiates, but increasingly used to denote both opiates and synthetic narcotics.

Paraesthesia is abnormal touch sensation, for example, burning or pricking, often in the absence of external stimuli.

Paresis is incomplete paralysis, a severe weakness rather than complete loss of use of a body part.

Pathological fractures occur when bone is weakened by disease, such as a tumour or osteoporosis.

Pel-Ebstein rising and falling fever occurs in Hodgkin's disease.

Pericardial effusion is a collection of fluid or blood in the pericardial space (smooth membrane surrounding the heart), caused by heart disease or cancer.

Peripheral neuropathy is a general term denoting functional deterioration in the body's outlying nervous system.

PET scan (positron emission tomography scan) results from a body scanner using particles with the mass of electrons, but a positive electric charge. A radioactive tracer is injected into the patient and shows up tumour activity in various parts of the body that may not otherwise be detected.

Phenothiazines are a group of major tranquillizers that also help in the treatment of psychoses.

Plasma cell neoplasms are abnormal growth of plasma cells.

Plasmacytoid differentiation relates to the plasma cells that are distinctive under the microscope to those around them and show cancerous changes.

Pneumocystis carinii pneumonia is a pneumonia that grows rapidly in the lungs of PLWHA and can occur in skin, eye, spleen, liver or heart.

Pneumonitis is inflammation of the lungs.

Postherpetic neuralgia is persistent burning pain and hyperaesthesia along the distribution of a cutaneous nerve following an attack of Herpes zoster, for example, in shingles.

Progressive multifocal leukoencephalopathy is a rare disease affecting the myelin sheaths (covering) of nerve fibres, and develops in immunosuppressed patients with AIDS.

Proprioception is the information provided by specialized sensory nerve endings in the joints monitoring muscle and tendon activity indicating joint positions in space.

Pruritis is itching, for example, uraemic pruritis is generalized itching associated with chronic renal failure and not related to other internal or skin diseases.

Psychostimulants are agents with antidepressant or mood-elevating properties.

Psychotropic drugs are used to modify mental activity, usually applied to drugs that affect the mental state.

Rhabdomyosarcoma is a malignant tumour of 'striped' muscle, such as that of the thigh or arm, mostly commonly seen in adolescents.

Sanfilippo's syndrome is associated with mucopolysaccharide, as it is a malfunction in these body proteins and metabolism. The skeleton may be un-affected, but severe cognitive and learning difficulties are likely to result.

Sarcoidosis is a disease of unknown origin with chronic inflammatory granulomatous lesions (new growth of tissue mass, not cancerous, which grows in response to the body detecting disease) in lymph nodes and other organs.

Sarcoma is primary cancer growth in soft tissue, connective tissue and bone.

Seroconversion illness is the change of a blood test from negative to positive indicating the development of antibodies in response to infection.

Sickle cell anaemia is a hereditary anaemia occurring in Afro-Caribbeans, characterized by crescent-shaped red blood cells, resulting in acute attacks of abdominal pain, ulceration of the lower extremities, severe pain in joints. It can be life-threatening.

Squamous cell carcinoma is a malignant tumour originating from an organ with a surface or lining epithelium of cells, for example, the bronchus or oesophagus.

Thalassaemia is a chronic anaemia occurring in Mediterranean families due to a specific gene influencing haemoglobin production.

Tuberculosis (TB) is a bacterial infection transmitted from person to person by an aerosol of organisms suspended in tiny droplets that are inhaled, e.g. breathing in near someone who has spat, coughed or sneezed out the infection.

Varicella zoster virus is the cause of chicken pox in children and shingles in adults.

Wiscott-Aldrich syndrome is a sex-linked genetic disorder occurring in male children, characterized by eczema, blood in stools and susceptibility to bacterial infections due to severe immunodeficiency.

Glossary – Abbreviations

ADC	AIDS dementia complex
ADLs	activities of daily living
AIDS	acquired immune deficiency syndrome
ALL	acute lymphoblastic leukaemia
AML	acute myeloid leukaemia
AMPS	Assessment of Motor and Process Skills
ARV	antiretroviral
BMT	bone marrow transplantation
CD4	protein structure on the surface of a human cell that allows HIV to attach, enter and thus infect the cell
CCD	Centre for Communicable Diseases
CML	chronic myeloid leukaemia
CMV	cytomegalovirus
CNS	central nervous system
COPD	chronic obstructive pulmonary disease
COPM	Canadian Occupational Performance Model
CT	computed tomography
EBV	Epstein-Barr virus
EEG	electroencephalogram
FIM	functional independence measure
GBM	glioblastoma multiforme
GI	gastrointestinal
HAART	highly active antiretroviral therapy
HAD	HIV associated dementia
HBV	hepatitis B virus
HD	Hodgkin's disease
HHV-8	human herpes virus 8
HIV	human immunodeficiency virus
HIVE	HIV encephalopathy
HPC	hepatitis C virus
HPV	human papilloma virus
HSV	herpes simplex virus
ICC	invasive cervical cancer

Occupational Therapy in Oncology and Palliative Care. Edited by J. Cooper
© 2006 John Wiley & Sons Ltd

KS	Kaposi's sarcoma
MAI	mycobacterium avium intracellular
MCD	multi-centric Castleman's disease
MM	multiple myeloma
MRI	magnetic resonance imaging
MTCT	mother-to-child transmission
NHL	non-Hodgkin's lymphoma
OI	opportunistic infection
PCNSL	primary CNS lymphoma
PCP	pneumocysitis carinii pneumonia
PEL	primary effusion lymphoma
PET	position emission tomography
PLWHA	people living with HIV and AIDS
PML	progressive multifocal leukoencephalopathy
POS	palliative care outcomes scale
RIC	Rehabilitation Institute in Chicago
SEIQoL-DW	Schedule for the Evaluation of Individualised Quality of Life
TB	tuberculosis
VZV	varicellar zoster virus
WIOM	Westcotes Individualised Outcome Measure
WISECARE+	Workflow Information Systems for European Nursing Care

Index

Lightning Source UK Ltd.
Milton Keynes UK

172518UK00001B/80/P